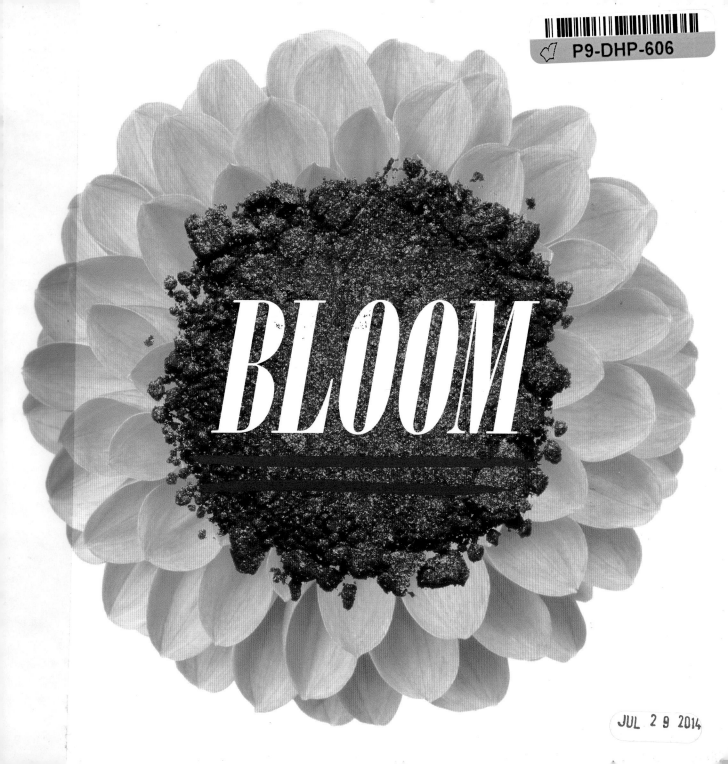

BLOOM

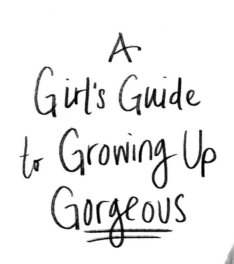

A
Girl's Guide
to Growing Up
Gorgeous

BLOOM

Carmindy

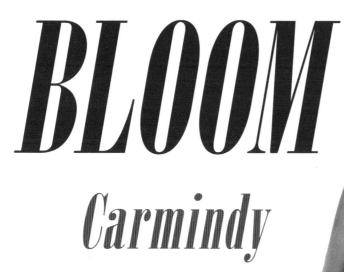

A PERIGEE BOOK

A PERIGEE BOOK
Published by the Penguin Group
Penguin Group (USA) LLC
375 Hudson Street, New York, New York 10014

USA • Canada • UK • Ireland • Australia • New Zealand • India • South Africa • China

penguin.com

A Penguin Random House Company

Library of Congress Cataloging-in-Publication Data

Carmindy.
Bloom: a girl's guide to growing up gorgeous / Carmindy.
pages cm
ISBN 978-0-399-16659-4
1. Teenage girls—Health and hygiene. 2. Cosmetics. 3. Beauty, Personal. 4. Face—Care and hygiene. I. Title.
RA777.25.C37 2014
646.7'2—dc23   2014010358

First edition: August 2014

PRINTED IN THE UNITED STATES OF AMERICA

10 9 8 7 6 5 4 3 2 1

Interior art: Flower collection © egal/iStockphoto; Isolated Daisy and Isolated Dahlia © Olaf Simon/iStockphoto; Daisy © Liliboas/iStockphoto; Dahlia, Rose, and Carnation © VIDOK/iStockphoto; Mallow © _Vilor/iStockphoto; Cornflower © AntiMartina/iStockphoto; Banana © EVAfotografie/iStockphoto; and Cucumber © nullplus/iStockphoto

Text design by Georgia Rucker

While the author has made every effort to provide accurate telephone numbers, Internet addresses, and other contact information at the time of publication, neither the publisher nor the author assumes any responsibility for errors, or for changes that occur after publication. Further, the publisher does not have any control over and does not assume any responsibility for author or third-party websites or their content.

Most Perigee books are available at special quantity discounts for bulk purchases for sales promotions, premiums, fund-raising, or educational use. Special books, or book excerpts, can also be created to fit specific needs. For details, write: Special.Markets@us.penguingroup.com.

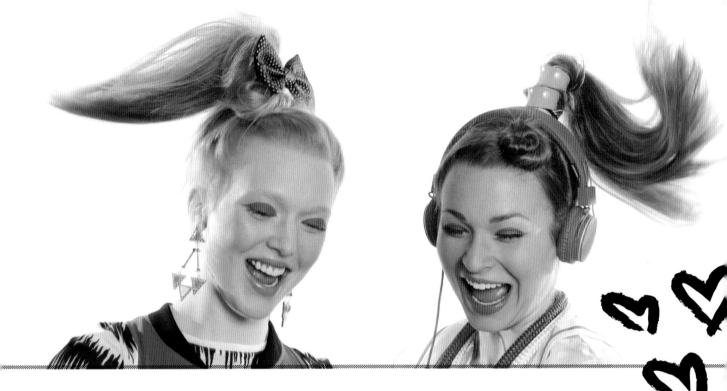

I dedicate this book to all the budding teenage beauties out there who have not yet realized that true beauty is the love and light in your heart, the clear, positive voice in your mind, and the celebration of your unique loveliness. Shine on, my fabulous flowers, never give up on loving yourselves, and always be your own beauty revolutionaries!

THERE ARE FLOWERS

everywhere,

FOR THOSE WHO

BOTHER TO LOOK.

—Henri Matisse

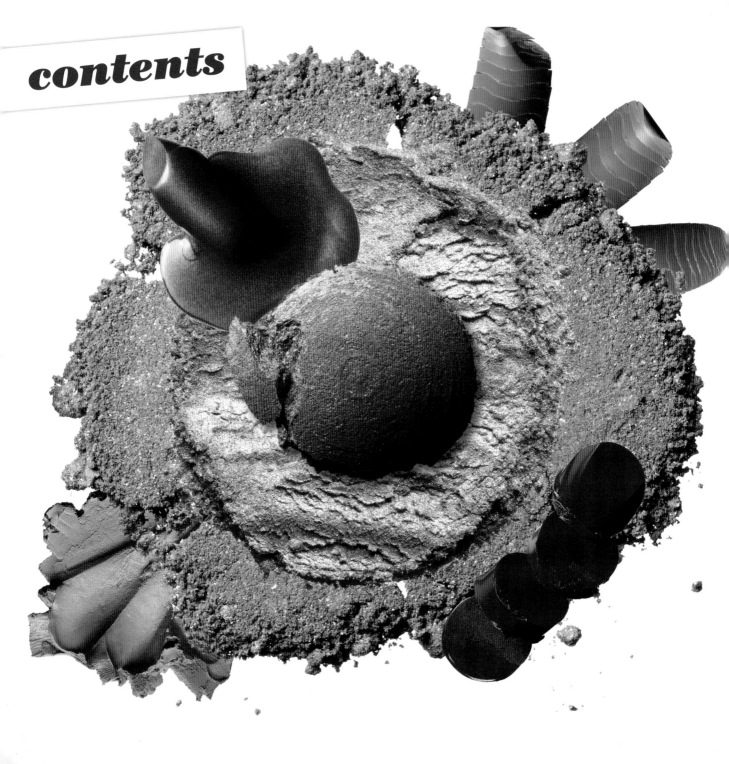

contents

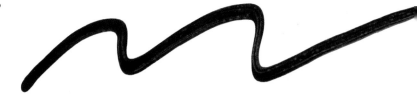

introduction

ARE YOU *READY* TO
Bloom
WITH ME?

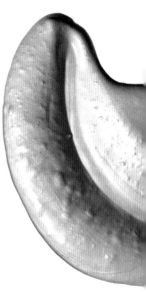

Have you ever heard the saying "A rose by any other name would smell as sweet"? Turns out that Shakespeare guy really was on to something. Ask any one of your friends what their favorite flower is. Now ask someone else. The more people you approach, the more varying answers you'll get. Some people think daisies are awfully sweet, and others are crazy about pansies. Tulips, daffodils, peonies . . . to borrow another famous expression, "Beauty is in the eye of the beholder." Everyone seems to have a completely different idea of what's considered gorgeous. Try to visualize what kind of flower you would be. Just pick your favorite and think about what makes it special. Think especially about what makes it stand apart from the other flowers. Just like each of us, there are seemingly unlimited variations of petals, each with different qualities that make them appealing. For example, roses are always lovely, but some people are especially drawn to honeysuckle, which may not be as showy, but its blossoms smell so sweet! Daffodils are especially charming to others, because their lovely goofiness makes them totally endearing. The famous female artist Georgia O'Keeffe painted many, many kinds of flowers—sometimes she focused on ones that boasted unique shapes; other times, specific colors inspired her—and she managed to highlight the idea that there is spectacular beauty in every bloom, if you look closely enough. Then remember how, like your flower, you are also super unique, whether it's the unusual color of your eyes or your adorable crooked smile. It doesn't matter if you're a delicate orchid or a wild cactus flower: This book is about celebrating them all. I see the beauty in each of you, and I want you to as well.

Here's another botanical quote for you: "The grass is always greener." I'm going to let you in on a juicy little secret that it took me years to learn. My curly brunette beauties out there, have you ever longed for super-straight blonde locks? Bold blue-eyed babies, do you think chocolate brown eyes are the ultimate accessories? It may sound crazy, but it's true on every level: Women of all ages seem to have this weird idea that if only they looked different, they would somehow feel better about themselves. Kinda silly, right? But it gets crazier: Sometimes I work with famous models and celebrities, and many times they're tall, have straight teeth, clear complexions—all the things the fashion magazines tell us is considered "beautiful." And here's the thing. They feel the same way. Tall, thin girls often say they wish they could be petite and curvaceous. Petite, curvy girls have spent more time than you could possibly imagine yearning to be more waifish and exotic. It seems everyone is sick with this envy disease.

The good news is, you don't have to play the compare-and-despair game. Our differences are what make us awesome! Walt Disney (I know you've heard of him!) said it best: "The more you are like yourself, the less you are like anyone else, which makes you unique." So stop that negative voice in your head right in its tracks and know that each and every one of our differences is actually what makes us beautiful. Once you fully understand that, you will begin to bloom like a flower in such magical ways that it will blow your mind. Embracing your own individuality with total confidence creates energy around you that people will want to emulate. Confidence is the product of self-love and it is truly what gives us the power to shine, to love, to laugh, to fall down and fail, and get up again to become better.

Ready for your inner flower power to grow? Any time you notice that you, a violet, are comparing yourself to the petunia next door, think of these thoughts as weeds in your garden—if they take root, they make it a little harder to see the beauty surrounding your particular petals. So put on your imaginary gardening gloves and yank those weeds right out of the ground. Let's get started!

chapter 1

PLANTING
THE
Seeds

True beauty comes from within. Here are a few ways to help you *own it,* ladies.

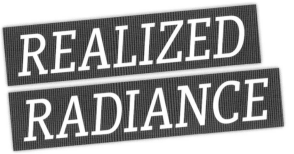

REALIZED RADIANCE

know it can be hard to really see yourself as beautiful in your teen years. These are the years when you're seeing a lot of changes in your body and appearance, and you're still trying to figure out who you are. It's not easy when we are constantly fed images of perfect models and flawless celebrities in the media who can make us feel insecure and inadequate because we don't look like them. Reality check: All of those seemingly perfect images you see in magazines and ads? It takes a team of people—from stylists to hairstylists, makeup artists, set designers, and more—to make sure the subject in the image *appears* to be flawless. What's more, I know you've heard of Photoshop and have probably used it for school or personal social media projects. Once the "perfect" picture is taken, then it gets fully Photoshopped! So obviously it's super unrealistic for anyone to compare themselves to that whole situation. Besides, how boring would it be if everyone looked the same and only one form of beauty mattered? It would be like everyone thinking only roses are beautiful and no other flowers mattered. Now honestly, my blossoms, I know *you* are way smarter than that. Now is the time to realize your radiance and change things up. You are a true beauty! Whatever you do, don't join Team Insecure and pluck out your petals. Take action and repeat after me: "I am beautiful and unique and we are all in this together." You may not believe it at first, but trust me, if you continue to repeat this mantra to yourself on a daily basis, slowly but surely, you will begin to recognize your inner flower power. Just try it (give it time!), and by continuing to focus on what makes you stand out in a positive way, you'll soon begin to bloom!

I wasn't always this confident myself. In fact, at times I was like total "Insecurity.com" when I was a teenager. I was a bit overweight, I had braces, and my mother permed my hair, which just accentuated my already round face. Kids in school called me all kinds of names, like "thunder thighs," "fatty," "basketball head," and "brace face." While I guess it kind of sounds funny now, at the time it hurt my feelings very much, and I totally stopped feeling pretty. I was bullied and dealt with the typical "mean-girls syndrome," and it began to really turn up the volume on that negative voice in my head— you know, the one we all have that tells us we're ugly or not good enough. I felt so unattractive and insecure that it started to limit my ability to pursue my hobbies and goals. I lived at the beach, loved the ocean, and had always wanted to join Junior Lifeguards and spend my days swimming, surfing, and learning lifesaving skills. The only issue was I had to be in a bathing suit every

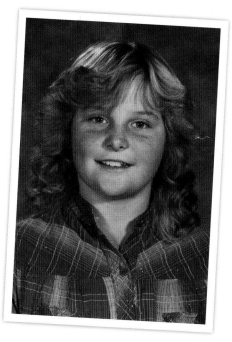

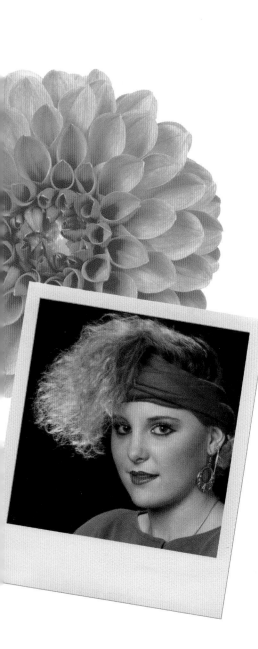

day, and all the teasing and taunting from the kids at school mixed with the loud, negative voice in my head stopped me from doing what I loved and I never joined up. How much does that suck?

I felt so bad after making that decision that I slowly realized I had to find a way to not place so much importance on what other people thought about me. Why should I allow others to control my destiny? Instead, I looked for ways to change my attitude. I realized that I was letting others influence my life, and only I could change it with more positive thoughts. I started practicing what I now call "Positive Mirror Mantras." When I would look in the mirror, the inevitable first thought I would have was, "I look fat," or, "I'm not as pretty as so-and-so." But I learned to instantly follow up those thoughts with positive ones, like, "I have pretty eyes," or, "I love my smile." At first, it was hard to truly believe the good comments I was saying to myself, but after doing it each and every day, I finally started a new pattern and broke the old one. Eventually, the Positive Mirror Mantras completely took over the negative voice in my head. I began feeling more and more confident, which led to feeling more sure of myself. That's how I was able to start redirecting my destiny. Once you believe in yourself, you start making decisions for you, because who cares what other people think? Try visualizing what hobbies and interests really make you happy and enthused, then acknowledge what—or who—is holding you back. Now push them out of the picture! Having confidence helped me get rid of those negative thoughts so that I could start pursuing my passions, and when you're operating from a positive place, you can do the same.

APPRECIATE, DON'T APPRECI-HATE

t takes loads of courage and strength to keep our heads up when we feel picked on, but when you do manage to stay cool, the outcome is so much sweeter. Instead of hating the girls who bullied me or feeling jealous—which is just more negativity that will bring your attitude down—I forgave them and, with compassion, wished them well in my heart. After all, most bullies are merely wrestling with their own insecurities. Positivity breeds positivity, and negativity breeds negativity. The choice, chicas, is yours. Inner happiness is not only beautiful, it radiates and it's contagious. Appreciate that growing pains can help you mature into a better person. So retrain your brain with Positive Mirror Mantras, let go of pain by forgiving and showing compassion for those who have hurt you, and start celebrating your unique beauty.

INSPIRATION NATION

Here's another cool way to do some "weeding" and start spreading the love. Start by giving what I call "Contagious Compliments" to others. Giving girls around you pretty props will not only make them feel good, but it will make you feel awesome too. For example, if you see a girl that has gorgeous hair, by all means, tell her so! If a friend of yours has nice eyelashes, then mention that to her. Contagious Compliments tend to spread like wildfire, and obviously, they are a hundred times more productive than tearing each other down. Be your own beauty revolutionary and start a Bloom movement of positivity in your own school or home by generously handing out Contagious Compliments, sharing Positive Mirror Mantras with your friends, and reminding others to celebrate their unique loveliness! Kind of like nutritious plant food, the more you spread

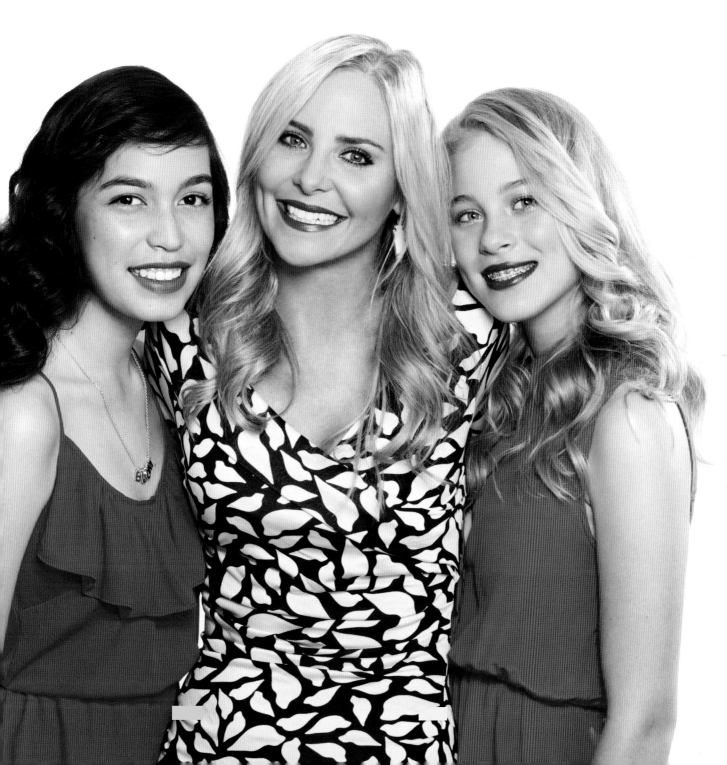

these small seeds of joy around, the more you encourage other flowers—and yourself—to grow healthy and proud.

Being a teen these days is tough, but I know you have the ability to nourish your self-esteem and bloom into a truly amazing person. Whenever you're feeling any doubt about it, simply revisit this chapter in order to remind yourself that you are not only a unique, beautiful flower, but that treating yourself and others with love and positivity will ensure an equally beautiful life.

Now my lovely blossoms, just like every great gardener has tools like spades and watering cans at her disposal, there are all kinds of beauty tricks and tips for you to choose from that can help you look and feel amazing. That's because, whether you've thought about it or not, inner and outer beauty are truly connected. We've been talking a lot about the foundations of beauty, and they are definitely in your heart, mind, and spirit. Without working on your Positive Mirror Mantras and your inner confidence, outer beauty is just plain superficial. But here's the cool thing that I love about my job: Using the art of makeup can actually work in tandem with your attitude to help you feel more confident on the outside, which can help you feel stronger on the inside too. It may sound silly, but think about how you feel on those days when you just kind of roll out of bed, don't bother

Without working on your Positive Mirror Mantras and your **inner confidence,** outer beauty is just plain superficial.

to brush your hair, throw on dirty clothes, and trudge off to school. You end up feeling kind of crappy, right? But what about those days (the first day of school or picture day come to mind!), when you take the time to pick out a cool outfit that you love and try your favorite hairstyle and perhaps a new lip gloss? You feel amazingly confident all of a sudden. You walk a little bit taller down the halls. That's because by making the effort to look your best, you're helping to project your inner beauty at the same time. And that's awfully powerful stuff. Consider this book your indispensable guide to marrying that inner and outer beauty. We'll cover all the basics and beyond like makeup 101, how to take a gorgeous Facebook pic, and the big one, what to do when you get a gigantic zit—*the horror!*—and how to help prevent them from happening in the first place. Let's get to it, ladies!

By making the effort to look your best, you're helping to project your inner beauty at the same time.

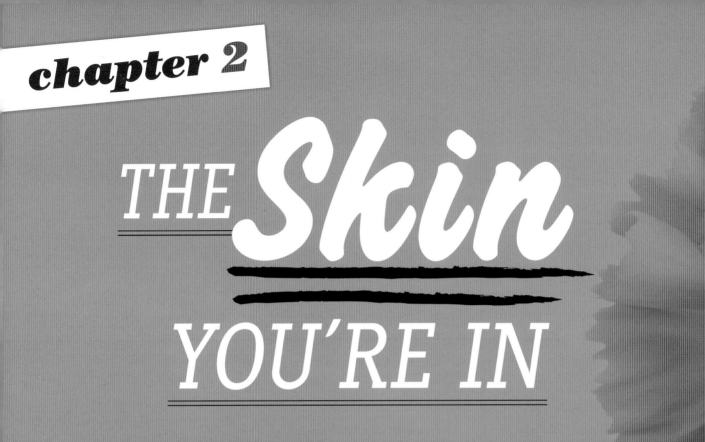

chapter 2

THE *Skin* YOU'RE IN

In order to create a beautiful painting, you need to start with a great canvas. That's why the most important step when it comes to your grooming routine is taking impeccable care of your skin. Getting into the good habit of cleansing, moisturizing, and protecting your skin each and every day will not only ensure that you're rocking an "It" girl glow, but by pampering it now, it will also stay beautiful for life. It's easy if you get into

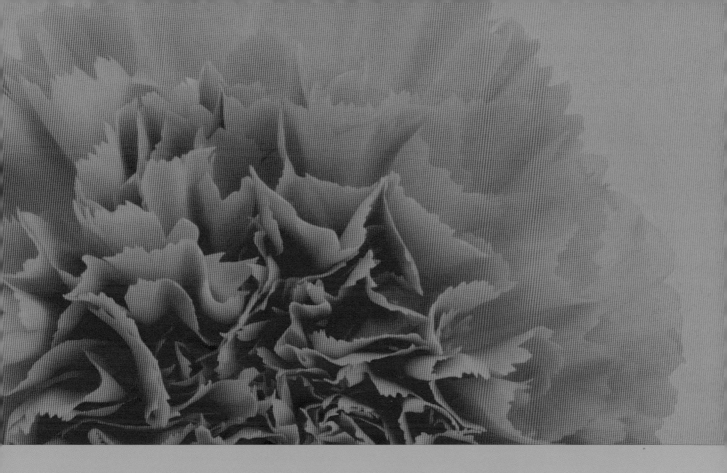

the same pattern with your skincare regimen as you do with, say, brushing your teeth. Twice a day, every day, make sure to cleanse, moisturize, and protect, and your complexion will thank you. Here's the best part: When your skin is in tip-top shape, you'll need less cosmetic products like foundation and concealer, so you can spend more time on the fun stuff like eye shadow and lip gloss!

CLEAN IT

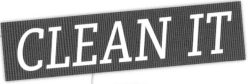

R ule number one when it comes to cleansing your skin: Never, ever go to bed without washing your face. Whether or not you wear makeup doesn't matter because after a long day, your skin has collected all kinds of gross dirt and grime that has built up and can lead to clogged pores, which can cause breakouts. Personally, I find that liquid face cleansers—there are tons of affordable drugstore versions from brands ranging from Cetaphil to Neutrogena—are the best way to achieve a squeaky-clean complexion. (That said, do yourself a favor and keep makeup remover and/or cleansing wipes on hand to remove stubborn cosmetics in a rush, though I do recommend following up with a liquid cleanser to eliminate any additional residue.) Let's talk about a few exceptions to this twice-a-day rule, though, based on skin type. Chances are, you have a pretty good idea of what skin type you are, but if you're still confused, follow these simple guidelines: If you notice scaly patches or general tightness, you're most likely dry. Combination skin means you have dryness, but sometimes you'll notice oily spots in the T-zone, which is the area from your forehead extending down through your nose and chin area. Oily skin is just what it sounds like: You may get greasy easily or notice you radiate a kind of natural "glow" that gets really shiny-looking at times. Sensitive skin needs a little extra care: You know you've got it if you flush easily or tend to have allergic reactions like redness or rashes from beauty products that contain fragrances or dyes. And finally, what the beauty industry often calls "normal" skin—perfectly balanced—is kind of a myth. What's normal anyway? Everyone's skin is completely different and unique!

Here are some general rules to go by:

● **YOU HAVE:** *dry or combination skin.* I know, I know, I said cleanse twice a day, but here's that exception I was talking about earlier: You can actually skip the cleansing step in the a.m. so that you'll retain your skin's natural moisture. At night, use a creamy cleanser that will help hydrate overly parched skin.

What's Up with Toner?

Toners can help refresh your skin after cleansing and before moisturizing. Toning is not a necessary step, but one that always feels good if you love that super, *super* clean sensation. Make sure to choose herbal toners that are alcohol-free: Harsh toners that contain alcohol can strip your skin of its natural oils, which can cause dry, flaky patches or an overproduction of oil, making troubled skin worse. I like to store my toner in the fridge and apply it to my skin with a cotton round, which refreshes my skin and tightens up pores before I put on my other products. To create a DIY toner, fill your bathroom sink with water. Add 2 cups of chilled apple cider vinegar. Start splashing your face multiple times; it may be a little stinky (or remind you of a school science project!), but trust me, ladies, you'll have a beautiful glow when you're finished. Finally, drain the sink and splash some cool, fresh water on your face to get rid of the vinegar smell. If you can't stand the aroma, try this: Steep one bag each of both chamomile and spearmint teas together in a large mug. Pour the resulting mix into a spray bottle, stick it in the fridge until it's cooled off, then spray onto your face after cleansing.

• YOU HAVE: *oily and acne-prone skin.* Wash your face morning and night, and try a foaming or gel face cleanser, as the lather will help wash away sebum (the yucky stuff that clogs pores) and won't leave a moisturizing residue behind. If you get oily throughout the day, use blotting sheets from the local drugstore to absorb the grease slicks, or try a mattifying gel to zap the shine. In a pinch, if you're at school and stuck with a too-shiny face and no blotting sheets in sight, a toilet seat cover will do the trick. Go to the restroom, rip off a piece of paper toilet seat cover, and press it to the oily area on your face to absorb the extra sheen. Hilarious, but it works.

• YOU HAVE: *sensitive skin.* Because it tends to irritate easily, make sure you stick to products that are fragrance-free. (If perfumes are added in your products, there's a good chance they will cause rashes or a burning feeling on your delicate mug. Just skip 'em!) Also, when you're washing your face, always rinse with cool water, which is more soothing and less irritating than hot. And skip the scrubs, as exfoliants can potentially make your skin angry. Finally, when it comes to trying new products, always spot-test makeup and skincare on a small area first to see if you have a reaction. If it feels good, then go for it!

• FOR ALL SKIN TYPES: Washcloths and buffing machines (like skin brushes) are antiaging accessories you don't really need until you get a bit older. The best face-washing tools you have are your own hands! Simply squeeze a quarter-sized dollop of cleanser into your clean palm, rub your hands together, and swirl the cleanser on to your wet face in circular motions for about a minute. Rinse it off with warm (never hot) water. Hot water can sometimes cause capillaries (tiny blood vessels) to break, which show up around your nose and cheeks in small, red, squiggly lines.

How to Exfoliate

Exfoliation is when you buff and polish away all the dead skin, extra sebum, and yucky muck that can collect on skin, causing blackheads and a dull complexion. Scrubbing off this "pileup" once a week will help create soft and glowing skin and prevent breakouts. At your age, steer clear of harsh exfoliants like glycolic and alpha hydroxy acids, which are too strong and irritating for young skin (unless you're having bad breakouts; see "The Big 'A'"). In fact, I suggest a much easier, not to mention cheaper, home remedy: Grab about a half cup of white sugar from your kitchen. When you take your usual shower or bath, simply pour out a handful, and rub it very gently on your face and body in circular motions. Do this once a week for a cheap and easy way to get a sweet complexion at home.

Poor Pores

Blackheads are those nasty little buggers that clog up your pores (usually on your nose or chin) and can make you feel like everyone is staring at them! Chances are, nobody notices them but you. The number one rule is to keep calm and carry on: Don't try to squeeze them, because it can not only create more breakouts; the pressure on your delicate skin can cause damage and even permanent marks. Instead, keep blackheads to a minimum by following a strict skincare routine. If you feel like they continue to be a major issue, use a pore strip (like the ones Bioré and other companies make) or a sugar scrub (see "How to Exfoliate") once every few days to help keep them at bay.

The Big "A"

It doesn't seem to matter what skin type you have: Thanks to hormones, chances are, like so many teens out there, you suffer from **acne**. Don't fret, my pets! You are so not alone. The first thing you need to understand is this is not forever, and you can absolutely, 100 percent get control over it. Rule #1 for acne is *do not pick*! Hear me, ladies? This will just cause scabbing and possible permanent scarring. Instead, switch to the right products. Choose cleansers, toners, and moisturizers that contain ingredients like salicylic acid, benzoyl peroxide, or sulfur. The key to getting acne under control and preventing new breakouts is total consistency in your acne-fighting skincare routine. That's why multistep kits like Proactiv have such a high success rate. These didn't exist when I was your age, but man, oh man, I could've used them! The idea is simple, and while buying a kit takes out all the guesswork, you can create your own as well. All you need is a simple cleanser containing salicylic acid, a toner containing a light glycolic acid, and a treatment to leave on overnight that contains benzoyl peroxide. I like to keep an acne spot treatment product that contains sulfur in the bathroom cabinet because it tends to be great for making an extra scary zit disappear overnight. (Yes, folks, acne can attack at any age!) But as long as you follow an antiacne regimen every day, twice a day, you should start to see a reduction in breakouts. If you've followed instructions closely for about six weeks—no cheating!—and still aren't seeing any results, then it's time to ask your parents if you can see a dermatologist who can help you explore other options.

MOISTURIZE IT

Think of moisturizing your skin now as insurance for the future: Your efforts to hydrate your complexion will pay off in a lifetime of supple and soft skin that radiates a beautiful glow. Apply your moisturizer in light, upward strokes to stimulate blood flow and to not drag the skin down. When blending moisturizer around your eye area, use your ring finger, which is the weakest finger, so you don't pull the delicate skin around your peepers. For oily or acne-prone skin, use an oil-free moisturizer; for normal to dry skin, you can use a basic, drugstore moisturizing lotion (no need to buy into fancy ingredients or buzz words like "antiaging"!). Combination girls who have trouble with extra shine in the T-zone can use an oil-free moisturizer along the "T" and a regular moisturizer on the sides of their face. For a fast two-in-one product, grab a moisturizer with a built-in sunscreen (also see "Protect It") so you stay moisturized and protected at the same time.

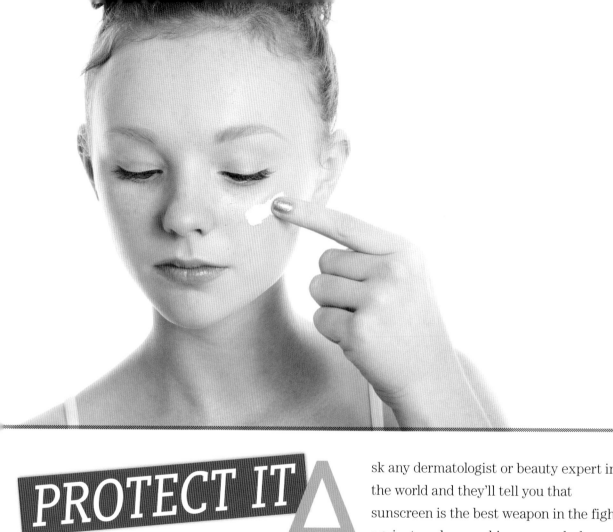

PROTECT IT

Ask any dermatologist or beauty expert in the world and they'll tell you that sunscreen is the best weapon in the fight against sunburns, skin cancer, dark patches, and premature aging, so, ladies, please take it seriously. Laying out and taking too much sun is bad for your skin, so promise me you won't do it! It also makes me crazy to hear how popular tanning beds can be among girls your age, and there's a reason why some states have banned them. Research shows that teens are in the highest risk category for overexposure to ultraviolet (UV) light, the harmful sun rays that can cause a lifetime of damage (um, like wrinkles, hello!). Even worse, too much exposure to UV light during your childhood years can greatly increase your risk of skin cancer later in life. So I really can't stress it enough: Wear your sunscreen every single day, no matter what! Get this: SPF is not just for summer. Dermatologists recommend wearing an SPF of at least 15 all year long—whether it's sunny or cloudy out—and reapplying throughout the day. I know remembering to do this is kind of annoying and not always practical in your busy day, which is where mineral powder sunscreens come in. These products are great because you can simply brush them on every few hours, and you get the added bonus of mopping up any excess shine. It's an awesome, must-have product to carry around in your backpack or purse. During the summer months (especially at the beach), you should bump up your sunscreen to an SPF 30 or higher. If you're out swimming, go for waterproof formulas and even then, you will need to reapply when you get out of the water. Nothing is worse than the dreaded sunburn, and tan lines look lame. (If you do accidentally get a tan line that you want to hide, blending on a little bronzer or self-tanner in the white area will help camouflage it.) And the last thing I'll say about sun protection is that you seriously cannot be careful enough. Because SPF can easily sweat off, always have a backup in the form of a good hat and sunglasses to help protect you when you're out enjoying the weather.

SPF is not just for summer.

BRONZE IT

It might look kind of weird if you're pale and then show up at school the next day looking like Malibu Barbie!

I get that some of you may be into the beachy bronze look. But I said it once, and I'll say it again: Never, ever, *ever* use a tanning bed! They are dangerous and should be illegal for people of all ages *everywhere* as far as I'm concerned. Nothing is pretty about skin cancer, and that's where you are headed if you cook yourself in a human microwave. If you really desire a tanned look, then you should know that it's never been easier to "fake the bake" using beauty products. Self-tanners and bronzers are totally safe, super easy to apply, and can look so pretty (plus, your skin will thank you!). To get the most realistic results, teens should use a gradual self-tanning moisturizer (Jergens makes a great range) that will build up your color over the course of a few days. After all, it might look kind of weird if you're pale and then show up at school the next day looking like Malibu Barbie! These gradual tan products come in shades from light to dark so you can choose a hue that more closely matches your natural skin tone. (If you are pale, trust me and go with the "Light" formula. Darker shades might turn out orange and give you the dreaded Oompa-Loompa effect!) The other thing I like about these gradual blends is that unlike some of the insta-tanners, they offer a more foolproof and forgiving way to get the glow, and you don't have to be a master blender, eliminating the chance of easy streaking. Here's how it works: Start off with smooth and even skin by exfoliating your face and body in the shower. You can easily do this with my favorite DIY face and body scrub made up of your cleanser and a handful of regular white sugar. Don't use store-bought sugar scrubs, as they contain oils that will leave a greasy film on the skin, preventing your self-tanner from absorbing into the skin. Next, when you get out of the shower, towel-dry and skip moisturizer so the product will absorb properly. Apply the gradual self-tanning moisturizer lightly but evenly to your whole body, working upward from your feet and ending with your face. Next, wash your hands right away with soap and water, using a washcloth. Then take the damp washcloth and gently buff over your elbows, wrists, knees, and feet in order to soften the areas where self-tanner tends to collect and become darker, which can cause streaks. This final step will help keep the color smooth and even-looking.

tip

When applying self-tanner to your face, you can also use a non-latex sponge to blend it on smoothly like you would a foundation. Make sure to cover your face, buffing it into the hairline, over the ears, and down the neck. This will ensure a streak-free, even, all-over glow to the face.

SPA
Sleepover!

It's so much fun to have a spa sleepover! Text your friends to come on over and join you for a pretty party. Here's the plan: Designate each girl to bring different beauty treats. For example, ask one friend to bring nail polish and tools for mani/pedis, have another bring her entire makeup box (have Q-tips and disposable applicators on hand so you don't exchange germs!), while another girl might bring headbands and ties for trying new hairstyles. You can also gather food ingredients in your kitchen to create DIY all-natural facial masks. Once you all get together, you can create a total beauty spa environment by mixing up and applying masks, watching YouTube how-to videos of cool new manicure styles, or practicing braided hairdos on each other. Don't forget to document the transformations on Instagram or Tweet new beauty tips and tricks you've learned so you can share with other teens out there. Here are my two favorite recipes for easy, made-in-your-own-kitchen spa sleepover facial masks.

The Super-Hydrating Banana Mask

> 1 medium banana
> ¼ cup plain yogurt
> 2 tablespoons honey

Add all ingredients into a blender and mix until smooth, then apply onto the face, avoiding eye area. Leave on for 20 minutes, then rinse off.

The Acne-Killing Cucumber Mask

> ½ cucumber
> 2 tablespoons dry oats
> juice of ½ lemon
> 1 tablespoon honey

Add all ingredients into a blender and mix until smooth, then apply onto the face, avoiding eye area. Leave on for 20 minutes, then rinse off.

FACE IT

Foundations and concealers are used to cover up imperfections on the skin like veins, spots, under-eye darkness, redness, zits, or any other discolorations. These kinds of products tend to be a must for older women, but teens can use them to simply conceal breakouts or redness. "Spot-concealing" is when you use a small, synthetic, fine-tipped concealer brush or non-latex sponge wedge dipped into foundation or concealer, and touch up the areas on the face you wish to conceal (as opposed to applying it to your entire face). Even if you have acne-prone skin, covering up your whole face with foundation and concealer will just make it look cakey and masked, so try to avoid it. To find the right shade of foundation or concealer for your skin tone, swipe on three shades that seem the closest to your natural color along your jawline, and look into a mirror in direct sunlight. (This is where department and drugstore samples come in handy.) The color that disappears into the skin is the right shade for you. Once you've spot-treated, the next step is to sweep on a sheer, translucent powder to set where you have applied the foundation and/or concealer so it will last all day. If you tend to get really oily throughout the day, the powder does the double duty of helping to keep your skin shine-free.

beauty note

Freckles are gorgeous, fresh, and most of all, fabulous! Never hate on your freckles and please, my darlings, never cover them up. Think of them as lovely little angel kisses and celebrate them. Don't forget: It's our differences that make us beautiful and unique!

BB (beauty balm) and CC (color corrector) creams are the latest high-tech formulas that blend sunscreen, skincare benefits, and coverage all in one. These kinds of products are an awesome quick fix for girls on the go who want to have a little more coverage and extra sun protection too. There's not too much difference between BBs and CCs except for claims and marketing speak, so choose one that seems to work best for your skin type and concerns and stick with it. BTW: These kinds of products can be a bit heavy at times, so for a lighter look, always apply over moisturizer, then use a non-latex sponge to blend and buff lightly into the skin.

The color that disappears into the skin is the right shade for you.

THE BOD SQUAD

Each girl is different and should start wearing deodorant as her body changes.

Taking care of the skin on your body is just as important as caring for the skin on your face. If you use a body moisturizer each day after you jump out of the shower, chances are you won't ever need to worry about dry or flaky skin. Try making your own customized body lotion by buying a large, unscented jug of body lotion, add in a few drops of your favorite perfume and a little shimmer dust, then shake it all up and apply. Violà! Fancy body lotion on the cheap.

Many teens tell me they're not quite sure when to start wearing deodorant. Each girl is different and should start wearing it as her body changes. The answer is really simple: If you begin to notice that you are sweating more or smelling a little musky throughout the day, then it's probably time to buy a stick of antiperspirant/deodorant and apply it each morning. Similarly, dealing with body hair can be a real pain for most teenagers, so deciding when to start shaving or bleaching is definitely a parent question. Ask your mom, dad, or guardian, and see what they have to say. Once they give you the go-ahead, then I think shaving is the best way to go for teenagers. For best results, under arms and legs should be lathered up with shaving foam first in a hot shower or bath. Never shave on dry skin or use cold water, which can cause abrasions and nicks. Choose a razor that has moisturizing strips, as they tend to glide over skin with ease, and shave from the ankles to just up over the knees and under the arms. If you have a lot of dark hair on your arms or face, try a bleaching kit (like Jolen, which comes with detailed instructions in the box) to lighten the hairs, as there is plenty of time to tackle more advanced techniques like waxing or lasers when you're older.

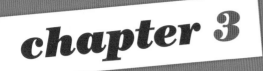

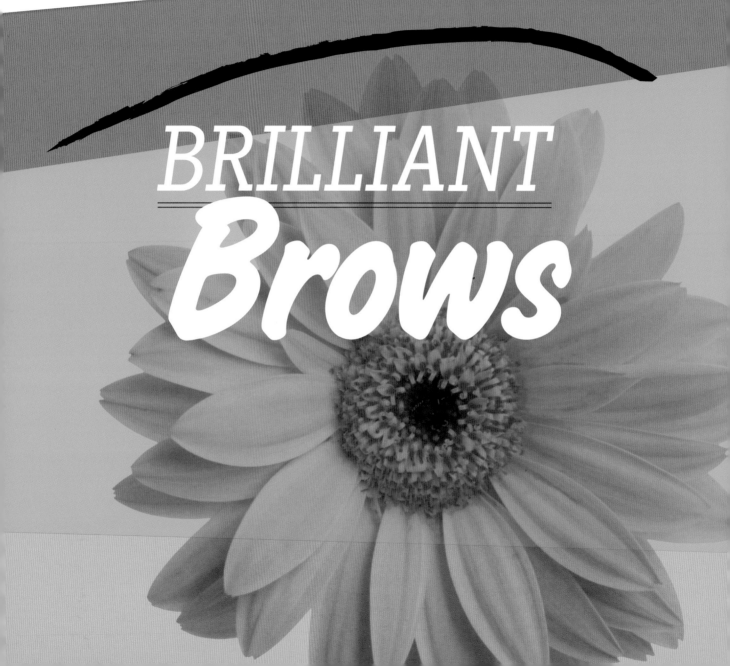

chapter 3

BRILLIANT
Brows

Well-groomed eyebrows can totally *make the face* by perfectly framing your pretty peepers. Too bushy and you risk looking like a wooly mammoth; too thin and it looks like you are really surprised . . . all the time. Finding the perfect, just-right brow for you depends entirely on looking at your natural brow shape and then practicing the proper grooming techniques. In this chapter, I'm going to show an easy way for beginners to learn how to groom their brows for a perfectly natural look.

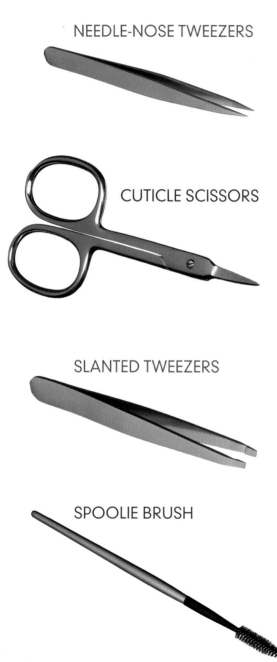

NEEDLE-NOSE TWEEZERS

CUTICLE SCISSORS

SLANTED TWEEZERS

SPOOLIE BRUSH

The most important tip for teens when it comes to getting brilliant brows is to always remember to stick to your natural brow shape as it is unique to your face. Do not ever try to re-create the shape of your own eyebrows to look like somebody else's, as that's where you get into trouble. You can really ruin your look, not to mention over-tweezing can cause some hairs to never grow back. I also don't like using brow stencils that you can find at beauty stores. It's like wearing someone else's bra: It's just not going to fit! So stick with your natural beautiful shape and just keep them polished.

The first step is to gather all the correct tools. You will need a pair of needle-nose tweezers, cuticle scissors, slanted tweezers, and a spoolie brush (those are the ones that look like mascara wands but are sold separately).

First, use the spoolie to brush the brows straight upward. If you notice any extra-long hairs that go up over your natural brow line, then snip them carefully with the cuticle scissors. If you happen to have brows that grow downward like many Asian beauties do, then brush them downward instead and snip away hairs that fall *below* the brow line.

Next, hold the slanted tweezers vertically along the side of your nose (1). Where the top of the tweezers hits your brow line is exactly where the hairs should begin. Pluck any stray hairs that grow between these two starting points of your brows. (If your brows don't extend that far, then leave them be!)

Now hold the tweezers again at the side of your nose and angle them so they cross the iris of your eye (2): Where the tweezers meet the brow line is where they should arch. Using the needle-nose tweezers (they're best for detailed precision and grabbing hard-to-reach hairs), pluck any strays that grow below this point.

Last, hold the tweezers along your nose and angle them so they cross the outside corners of the eyes (3). This is where the brow should end. Pluck any stray hairs that grow beyond this point.

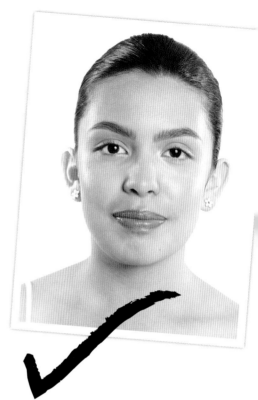

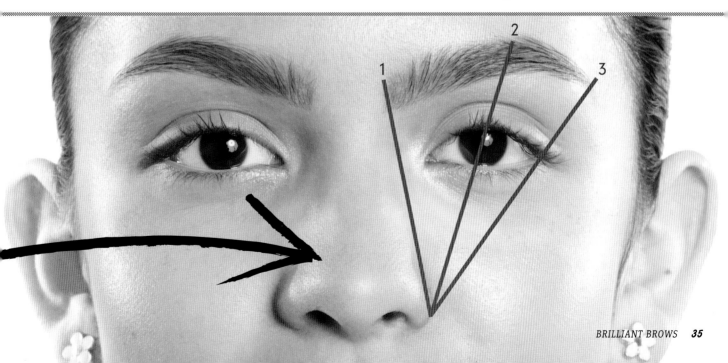

HOW BROW MAKEUP WORKS

There are so many mistake-fixing brow correctors out there, from powders to pencils to gels and pens, but hopefully, as a teen, you can avoid going crazy with all the overwhelming options and leave your brows free to do their thang. That said, here are a few guidelines when it comes to the occasional cleanup. (And a note on brow products: There's really no need to spend a lot of money on these, so check out super-cheap options available at almost any drugstore.)

If you have a gap or brows that seem to fall a bit short, the right product can fix the issue in a flash. For a very obvious "bald spot," a simple brow pencil is the way to go. Just make sure the tip is sharp and pointed so you can lightly feather in the area with tiny little strokes. A brow pen can do the trick as well, and many these days are waterproof, so they'll stay put all day long.

For curly or unruly arches that don't seem to stay in place, a tinted brow gel is your new best friend. Simply brush the gel over your brows and, like a good hairspray, it will hold them in place all day. For brows that tend to

> There's really no need to spend a lot of money on these, so check out super-cheap options available at almost any drugstore.

be super blonde, I'd recommend to just embrace your natural unique, ethereal look. If you really just can't live with them, try applying a little brow powder, which will darken them slightly but will still look natural.

Beware of Brow-arexia

There is a crazy skinny-brow epidemic going around among young ladies that is threatening the natural beauty we possess. Too many girls are yanking, plucking, pulling, and waxing off their brows in some crazy attempt to mimic the look of another person's brows. Know this: If you tweeze your brows too thin, it not only looks weird but, worse, they may never grow back if you keep it up! Just ask your mom or grandma: They might even have their own story about how over-tweezing can cause permanent brow loss. Extra-skinny brows can also make you appear older (but not in a good way), so it's best to stick to a natural look and go easy with the tweezy, got it? If you have already over-tweezed, please, I beg you, let them grow back. You can use a brow pencil or powder to fill them in while you're waiting to get them back into a full, healthy shape. Remember, it's like growing out your bangs, so be patient. Whatever you do, just don't be a pluck-aholic!

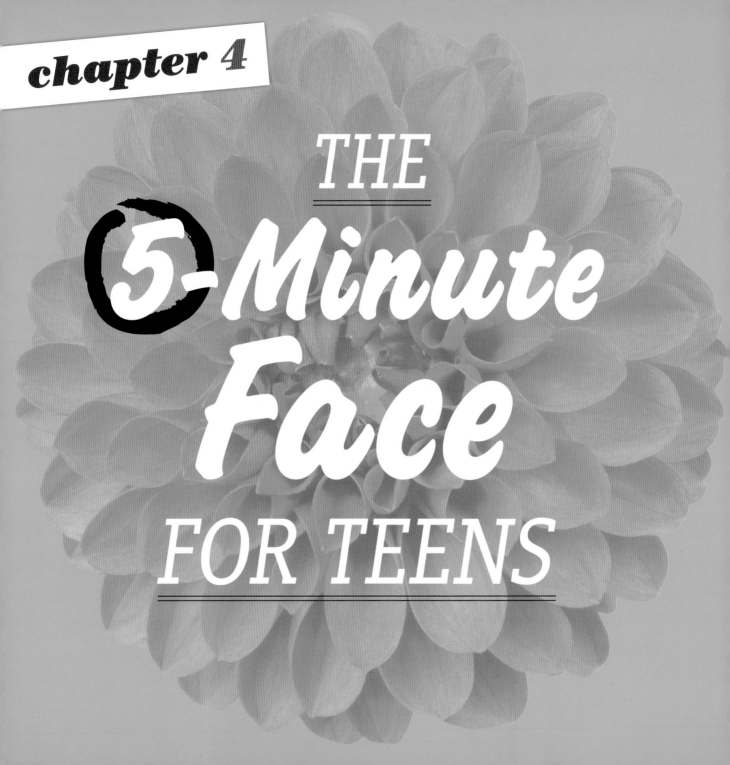

chapter 4

THE 5-Minute Face

FOR TEENS

Most pretty young flowers like you don't need a multistep makeup routine each day to truly bloom. Besides, you have a million better things to do than to spend hours in front of the mirror! Instead, play up your unique, individual beauty in just a few simple steps with my "5-Minute Face for Teens" technique. I want to teach you how to enhance your natural beauty in a quick and easy way so you will shine like the perfect little goddess you are in a flash. I get it: You have a busy social schedule, so this six-step technique will ensure you can stay on top of your game in a clean way that even your parents will love!

Tools

> small-tipped synthetic concealer brush

> foundation or concealer (in your ideal shade)

> small powder brush

> translucent powder

> Carmindizing highlighting cream

> Q-tips

> powder blush

> large blush brush

> black or brown mascara (bright colors optional!)

> lip gloss or tinted balm

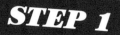

Even out your lovely skin by using the small concealer brush to spot-conceal any blemishes, redness, or darkness with concealer or foundation. To cover red areas (like around the nose), a small amount of foundation is your best bet. For blemishes that need a bit more coverage, concealer (it has a bit more pigment in it) is definitely the way to go. Remember to not overdo it as your freckles, skin tone, and natural texture should always, but always shine through.

STEP 2

Apply a light dusting of translucent powder to set the makeup you have just applied so it will last all day and not slip and slide around your face. You can use a loose translucent powder with a small powder brush to apply it lightly; a large powder brush will apply too much powder. If you are using a pressed powder, use a puff to gently *tap* the powder on your skin; rubbing it across the skin will just erase the spot-concealer you applied beforehand.

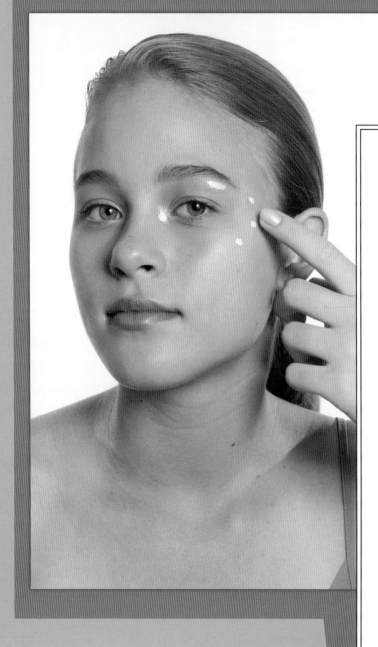

Time to Carmindize! Carmindizing is using a highlighting cream to bring light and illumination to your face. When you apply it in three key places—under the brows, on the inside corners of the eyes, and on top of your cheekbones—this technique gives you a lit-from-within glow that looks truly magical. When blending it under the brows, use your ring finger and blend it across the entire brow bone. For the inside corner of the eyes near the tear duct area, use a Q-tip to dab a bit of highlighter in this area, and then blend it in with your finger as needed. For the tops of the cheekbones, use your pointer and middle fingers to blend on the highlighter, starting from the tops of the cheekbones and blending back to the hairline. You can also blend a little at the temples for a more intense glow.

STEP 4

In order to define your eyes, all you need to do is to sweep one coat of mascara onto the top lashes only. This is all your perfect peepers need to stand out when you're in a rush. For a more playful look, try colored mascara like blue, green, or purple instead of basic brown or black.

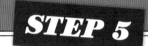

STEP 5

Quickly swirl on a flush of your favorite subtle blush shade (the hue your cheeks naturally flush) to the apples of your cheeks (the round part that forms when you smile) using a big, fluffy powder brush. Using this type of brush will generously hug the apples of your cheeks in one easy sweep.

Last but not least, play up your lips with a slick of gloss or tinted lip balm—you could go for a natural look (one shade darker than your normal lip color) or a more playful trendy hue—and you are ready to roll. Polished perfection!

practice

If you're feeling a little unsure about how to do this, check out my 5-Minute Face video selfie at carmindy.com and try it alongside me. The more you practice applying your "5-Minute Face for Teens," the more you'll notice yourself become even faster and more precise. Honestly, it's so quick and easy that you can do this on the way to school to save even more time. Now get going!

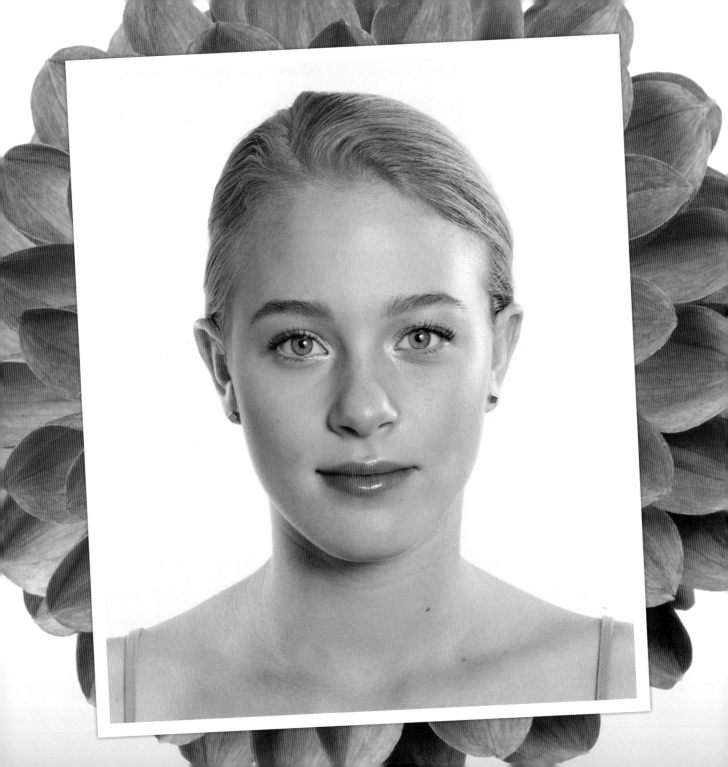

Touch-Ups

There is a time and a place for makeup touch-ups. A little etiquette goes a *very* long way! Maybe this sounds old-fashioned, but I truly believe that you should never, ever whip out your compact and reapply your makeup in public. I personally think it's bad manners, as you should be paying attention to your company, not your face. (Same goes for checking texts at the table!) Excuse yourself to the ladies' room (as you, my dear, are a *lady* after all), and then reapply your powder, gloss, or whatever you may need. If you do get stuck at a table and can't leave and feel like your lips are getting really dry, try my sneaky lip trick: Under the table, casually pull out your lip product from your purse or backpack and dab some of it on your pinky finger. Then when nobody is looking, simply bring your arm up, rest your chin on your hand, and quickly swipe your pinky finger across your lips and press them together. Violà! Moist lips and you maintained your classiness! Very James Bond, wouldn't you agree?

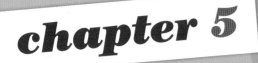

chapter 5

ANGEL *Eyes*

When it comes to your pretty peepers, all shapes and colors of eyes are beautiful. No matter if they are small, large, wide-set, close-set, eyes really are the center of your flowering beauty. And the best part? Playing up your eyes with makeup and learning how to showcase them in different ways is the most fun way to make a statement. For many of you teen beauties, eye makeup seems super hard to learn. There's no question: With so many different looks to try and products out there, it can sometimes seem downright intimidating! And some of those crazy how-to makeup tutorials on YouTube look overdone and ridiculous. Trust me, ladies, you don't have to try so hard. Less is definitely more! As trends come and go and you begin to get more comfortable using eye makeup, you'll get more confident in terms of mastering more advanced looks. For now, I want to concentrate on some easy techniques that will create a fresh, pretty, more natural look. These basic eye looks will not only work on all of you stunning teens (no matter what shape of eyes you may have), but they're also age-appropriate so you will never look like a hot mess.

PUT IT IN NEUTRAL

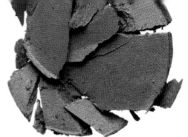

The most basic and simple look is the neutral eye. It's a great way for beginners to play with more than just mascara, and it will also teach you how to blend eye shadows together. Once you master this look, you can branch out with more intricate looks.

Tools

> dark brown eyeliner pencil

> Q-tips

> Carmindizing highlighter

> lid eye shadow brush

> midtone eye shadow (soft brown if you're fair skinned ranging up to dark brown for dark skin)

> mascara

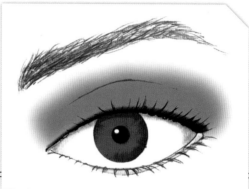

Start by drawing a thin line of the brown eyeliner across the upper lash line, getting as close to the roots of the lashes as possible. Next, use the Q-tip to smudge the liner for a soft effect. Dab on your Carmindizing highlighter underneath the brows, across the brow bone area, and on the inside corners of the eyes. Next, use the lid eye shadow brush to sweep the midtone shadow across the eyelids from where you applied the liner to just up and over the crease or midway point of the lids where it meets the Carmindizing highlight. Last, finish with mascara on the upper lashes only.

Opposites Attract

Want a quick way to make your unique eye color stand out? Think opposites. If your eyes are blue, you can use a brown shadow or eyeliner to make them totally mesmerizing. If you have a green-eyed gaze, purple shades can really make them pop. Brown eyes are especially bold when paired with blues, and hazel eyes look gorgeous next to green.

Mascara Styles

Choosing the right **mascara** is easy once you learn what shade to buy. Black is a great choice no matter your skin tone or hair color because it makes a real impact. If you have fair skin and light hair, brown mascara will create a more natural look. Colored mascara is also a fun way to play up your eyes if you're not quite ready for eyeliner and eye shadows yet.

Fun with Falsies

Have you ever wanted to try **false eyelashes** on for size? As intimidating as they seem, it's actually super easy if you follow my little snip trick. Hold a pair of drugstore falsies, then snip them in half with a pair of cuticle scissors. Grab the smaller section (the side with the shorter lashes), then squeeze a dab of eyelash glue onto the back of your hand, and lightly drag the seam of the lash through the glue. Give the glue a few seconds to get a bit tacky, then hold and press this half lash at the outer corners of your own upper lash line. This a simple way to handle and apply lashes, and by using only half, they'll look very natural. Lastly, sweep on mascara to blend the real with the fakes for a fabulous full lash look.

NEON DELIGHT

Another cool thing about playing with makeup as a teen is you can get away with a lot! Have fun with it. Bright, bold colors are all the rage, which is really awesome for a party or special occasion. Blue, green, purple, orange, neon, and even glitter eyeliners can be swept on fast and give you a fab look in a flash.

Tools

> pencil sharpener

> eyeliner pencil in bright shade of your choice

> mascara

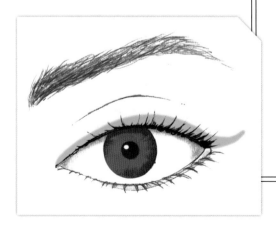

To easily line the eyes, always sharpen your pencil first so the line will be precise and the pencil tip will be clean. Start by sweeping the tip of the liner from the inside corner of the eye along the upper lash, ending at the outside corner, close to the roots the whole way so there is no gap of skin showing between the lashes and the liner. If your eyes are small or close-set, begin lining them at the center point of the lid. If your eyes are large or wide apart, then start at the inside corners of the eyes. (Remember this eyeliner rule whenever doing any of the looks in this chapter.) When using an extra-bold liner, skip any additional eye shadow and just sweep on black mascara along the upper lashes only. By keeping the rest of your makeup minimal, you'll look modern and fresh, not cray-cray!

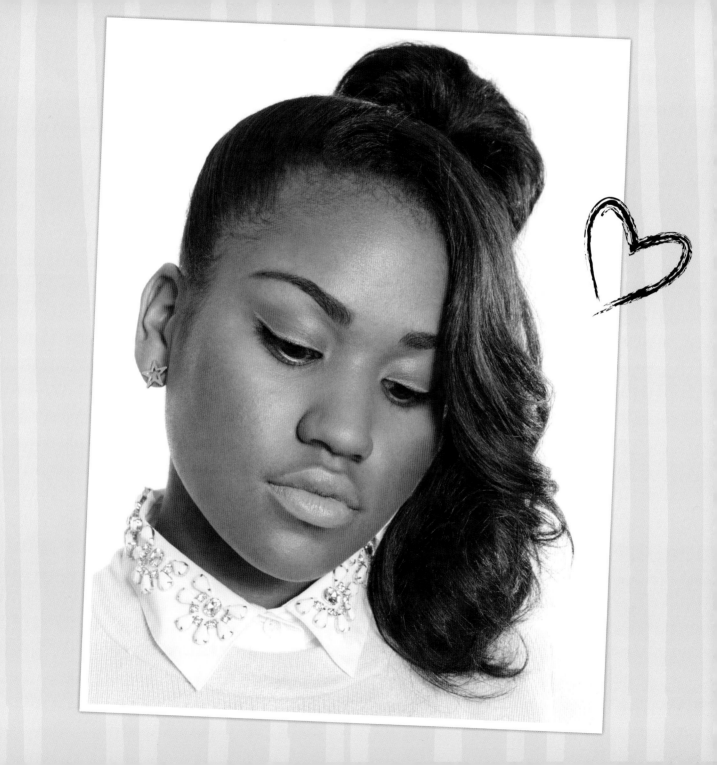

THE MERMAID GAZE

This is a fun way to play with glitter and iridescent colors. If you keep the rest of your face neutral, it will look super cool and can be worn no matter what color skin tone you have. Just remember, the darker your skin is, the deeper the shades you should choose. Save this kind of fantasy look for a special occasion; it's a bit much for, say, school.

Tools

> teal eyeliner pencil

> lid eye shadow brush

> shimmering turquoise eye shadow

> angle brush

> dome-shaped (crease) eye shadow brush

> mauve eye shadow

> double-ended highlighting eye shadow brush

> iridescent Carmindizing powder highlighter

> mascara

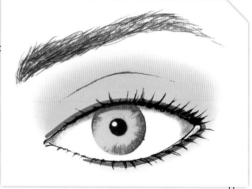

Start by lining the upper and lower lash lines with the teal eyeliner pencil. Next, use the lid eye shadow brush to sweep the shimmering turquoise eye shadow across the lids, and use the angle brush to sweep it along the lower lash line over the eyeliner line. Using the dome-shaped brush, sweep a hint of the mauve eye shadow across the eyelid crease. Use the larger side of the double-ended highlighter brush to apply the iridescent Carmindizing powder highlighter directly on the brow bone area. Use the smaller side of the brush to apply it on the inside corners of the eyes. Finish with a coat of mascara on top and bottom lashes.

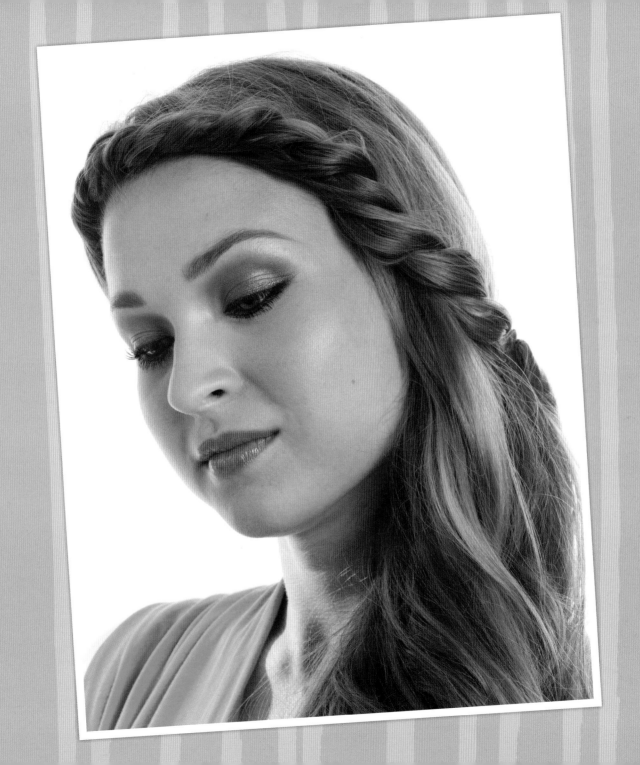

CAT EYES

The retro cat eyeliner technique has been cool since the '60s, yet the look is definitely here to stay. Wielding a liquid liner can be a total pain and many teens wish they could get it right but instead wind up majorly frustrated. No need to fret, my feline friends: It's a snap if you know a few secret cat eye tips. Liquid eyeliner comes in many forms, from tapered brush applicators to liquid eye lining pens or the pots of gel liner formulas. Whichever one you choose, trust me, you will master the perfect cat eye by using the following rules.

Tools

> pencil sharpener

> black eyeliner pencil

> liquid eyeliner

> small-tipped synthetic concealer brush

> foundation

> mascara

The secret to getting the perfect cat eye every time is, well, patience. Don't try this look in a hurry, especially if you've never attempted it before. Set up some good lighting, give yourself a license to chill, and you will eventually sweep on cat-winged liner like a pro. The first step is to create a stencil outline on your eye with the black eyeliner pencil. Sharpen your pencil, then draw a straight line along the upper lash line, creating a "stenciled" line for the liquid liner to trace. Next, sweep the liquid liner on top of the pencil, going over the pencil line from the inside corner to the outside corner, then flipping it up and outward in a small wing at the ends. You can also slightly tug at the outer corners of the eyes with your finger to make your lids more taut, which will make it easier to apply the wings. Now stand back and look into the mirror. If the wings aren't even, simply dip your small-tipped concealer brush into a little foundation and clean up the edges. The brush will act like a little magic eraser so you can fix it and not have to totally start over. Finish with mascara on the upper lashes only.

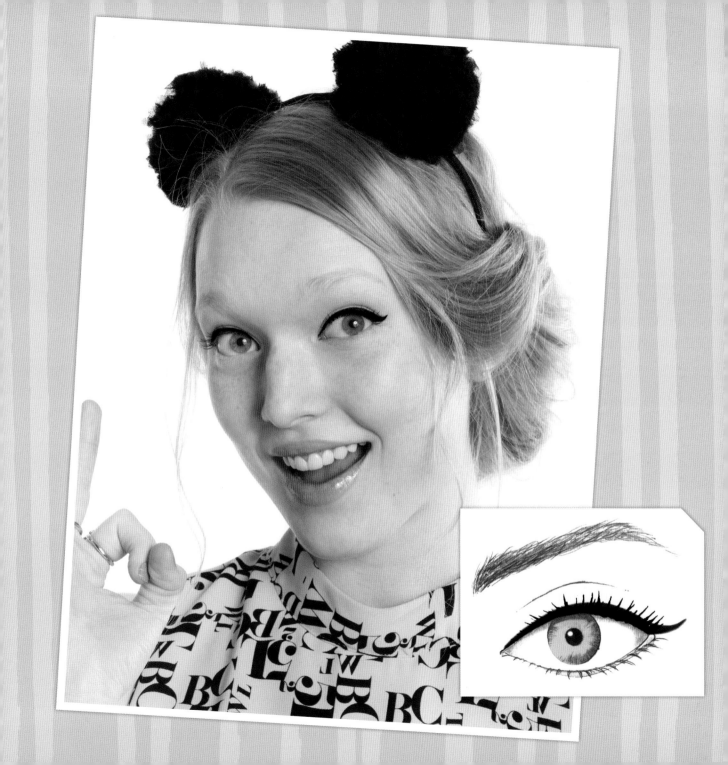

SMOKY EYE LIGHT

The classic smoky eye is uber popular, but you can end up looking like you have two black eyes if you're not careful. Using this "light" version, you can look like a cool teen, not a drag queen. It's all about the gradation of color and pairing it with a natural-looking lip for balance.

Tools

> pencil sharpener

> black eyeliner pencil

> lid eye shadow brush

> slate gray eye shadow

> angle brush

> dome shaped crease brush

> midtone granite eye shadow

> double-ended highlighting eye shadow brush

> Carmindizing powder highlighter

> mascara

Start by lining the top and bottom lash lines with a sharpened black eyeliner pencil. You can also line the inside (water line) of the eyes if you have medium or large eyes, but skip this step if your eyes are on the smaller side. Then, using the lid eye shadow brush, blend on the slate gray eye shadow across the lids, from where you applied the black eyeliner, blending up to the midway point, or crease, of the eyelids. With your angle brush, blend a bit of the slate shadow along the lower lash line. Next, grab your dome-shaped eye shadow brush and sweep the midtone granite eye shadow across the crease. With the larger end of the highlighting brush, apply the Carmindizing powder highlighter under the brows on the brow bones, and with the smaller end of the highlighting brush, apply it on the inside corners of the eyes. Lastly, sweep on a healthy dose of mascara on the top and bottom lashes.

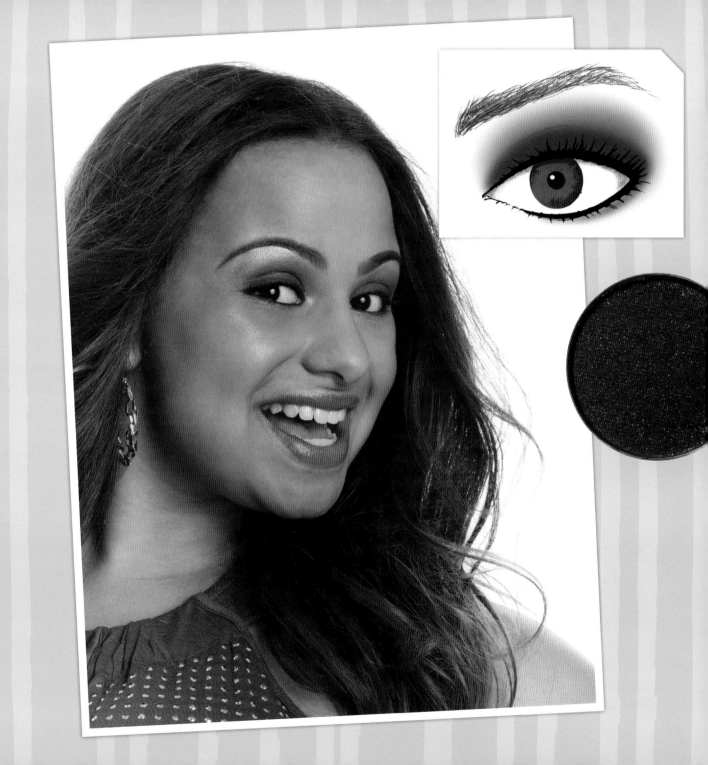

How to Curl Your Lashes

If you have straight eyelashes, a lash curler will curl them up for a wide-eyed, flirty look. My favorite lash curler on the market today is the corner lash curler because it lends you so much precision. This smaller tool allows for each lash to be curled in sections, whereas the larger, more traditional curlers can sometimes miss lashes, not fit the eye shape, and can just be hard to manage overall. Always curl bare lashes instead of mascara-coated ones, as the latter increases the risk of breakage or ripping them out. Start at the inside of the lash line, and gently crimp the base of the lashes. Hold for a few seconds, then move upward (just a tick!) on the lash and repeat. Slowly continue this method, moving across the lid and repeatedly curling until you reach the outer corners. Immediately apply mascara to hold the curl in place.

No More Smudges

Nothing sucks more than having "raccoon eyes" after creating a flawless eye look because your makeup has slid down your face by day's end. It's the worst! There are a few quick fixes for ensuring your handiwork stays in place all day and night. If you have oily lids, and cream or powder shadows always seem to turn into a creasy-greasy mess, then try applying a mattifying gel as a primer first to control oil. If you are doing a more dramatic eye, like a Smoky Eye Light, you can guarantee your blending will stay put by first covering the eyelids with a little foundation and powder, as this will give the shadow something to adhere to. Not only will the colors stay true but you'll be smudge-proof. In general, when lining eyes, opt for waterproof formulas and choose mascaras that are either waterproof or "tube technology" formulas. Tube technology is a type of mascara that coats each individual lash with a polymer that doesn't smudge like a traditional mascara formula does, but washes off much easier than a waterproof formula would.

quick fix

If you apply glitter eye shadow and some of it falls off onto your face, simply grab a piece of tape and press it on top of the glitter specks. When you peel it off, the glitter comes with it.

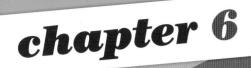

chapter 6

YOU'RE SO
Cheeky

Smile, ladies! Using blush to enhance your cherub cheeks is the quickest way to wake up the face, warm up your complexion, and best of all is a totally subtle way to play with makeup that's super age-appropriate. If you use cheek color the right way, you can achieve a soft, romantic look that is healthy, natural-looking, and surrounds your smile with sweetness.

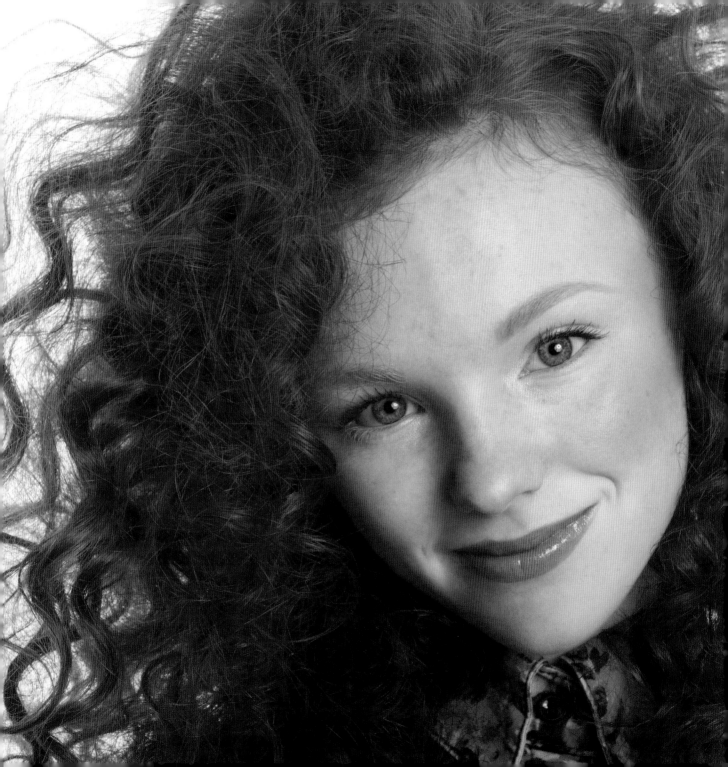

How to Find the Right Blush Shade for You

Here's the absolute easiest way to find the most perfect, Mother Nature–approved color of blush that will always look great on you. Next time you exercise, run right over to the drugstore! You are looking for a shade that matches the subtle hues of pink or red that your skin flushes to naturally. That said, there is always room to play. Light and pale skin tends to look pretty in most shades of pink and peach. Medium skin tones look amazing in rose and coral hues. For dark skin, the brighter and bolder the better, so look for reds and golden bronzes. If you have acne-prone skin, then stick with matte finish blushes, meaning they don't have any shimmer in them, so they won't highlight any raised surfaces on the skin.

BLUSHING BEAUTIES

No matter what type of blush you choose to apply, the golden rule is to apply the color to the apples of your cheeks, or, the round areas that look more prominent when you grin. To find the "apples," simply smile big: The round, fleshy part of the cheek is the exact spot where you'll want to sweep on the color. The "two-finger rule" can also help when you're trying to locate exactly where to place the blush. Two fingers' width away from your nose is where you begin and two fingers' width under your eyes in how high you should go. No matter if you have round cheeks, flat cheeks, high cheeks, or low cheeks, there is always room to play with a pop of color and bring them to life. I do not want to hear you complaining that you have chubby cheeks or that you have no cheekbones! The way your cheeks look is just one more way that you're beautifully unique, and besides, a healthy flush of color looks amazing on everyone.

Apply blush as the very last step of your makeup routine, because chances are you will only need a hint of tint on those cheeks. Less is more! Try to put your blush on in natural daylight or at least right next to a window if possible. Artificial light can be deceiving, and you may use too much. Correct application should look like you're naturally flushed.

> The way your cheeks look is just one more way that you're **beautifully unique, and** besides, a healthy flush of color looks amazing on everyone.

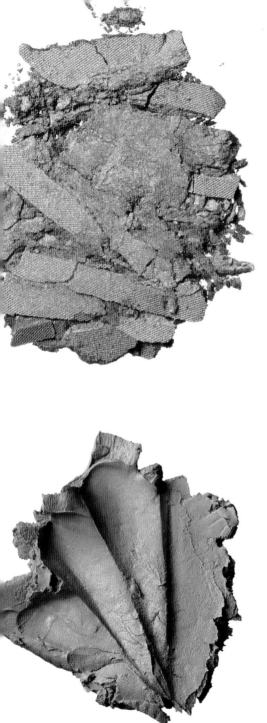

• POWDER BLUSH: These formulas are the most common type and work on most skin types, but tend to be best for oily skin because they won't slip and slide on your face. To apply, use a big, fluffy powder brush instead of a traditional blush brush or the ones that often come free with the product. This is because those smaller, old-school blush brushes tend to pick up too much product and deliver it in a concentrated way on the skin, making it harder to blend. You definitely don't want to look like a circus clown! It may cost extra, but you might be surprised by the quality of inexpensive brushes you'd find at the drugstore. Just dip the big fluffy brush in the product, tap it against your hand to let any excess blush fall off, then gently sweep it on the apples of your cheeks for a soft, natural-looking flush. If you feel like you have applied too much, simply use a little translucent face powder to sweep over the top to tone it down.

• CREAM BLUSH: Because these types of formulas can help add moisture to the skin, they are ideal for dry-skinned girls. There are a few reasons why I love, love, love cream blush and you should too: Because the product just melts seamlessly into skin, it gives off a hyperrealistic-looking color. It's also super easy to apply because all you need are your fingers. Just tap the tips of your index and middle fingers into the cream blush, then apply directly to the apples of your cheeks in circular motions until it blends in perfectly. If you apply too much, you can dip a non-latex sponge into a little liquid foundation and buff over top to lighten the look.

• **CHEEK STAINS:** Gals with "normal" skin—that is, not super dry or oily—should totally check out cheek stains for a stay-put pretty flush. These usually come in both gel or balm forms and are great for those busy days when you're running from classes to after-school practice and you can't be bothered to touch up. Stains should be applied with fingers or a sponge, and the key is that you want to blend them in quickly so the stain doesn't set before it's blended. Again, you can use the sponge trick (see "Cream blush") to even out any parts that look blotchy.

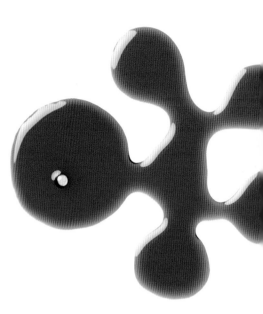

• **BRONZERS:** I love bronzer because it gives you that healthy, outdoorsy look without a tan (which you promised me you'd never, ever do, remember?). Bronzers come in all shapes and sizes from powder form to gels that are squeezed out of a tube, but the key is staying in the lighter, rosy-bronze color zone if you're pale and more robust golds and ambers for darker skin. Teens with dry skin can blend on a cream bronzer using fingers or a non-latex sponge wedge, while girls with oily skin do better with a powder bronzer and a big, fluffy powder brush. Combo-skinned ladies can use either. The right way to apply the bronzer is in a C formation on the face, starting at the temples,

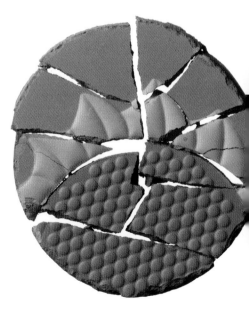

Again, you **don't** want to look like an Oompa-Loompa!

sweeping along the sides of the face, and ending under the cheekbones. Then, very lightly sweep any leftover color softly across the forehead, nose, and chin. The bronzer is concentrated around your face in that C, hugging it with a sun-kissed glow, and the center of your face is lighter, which will keep you looking natural and not overdone. Just don't make the mistake of putting it all over your face. Again, you don't want to look like an Oompa-Loompa! (Not a good look.)

My technique will ensure that you will never look muddy or dirty; more like beach babe perfection!

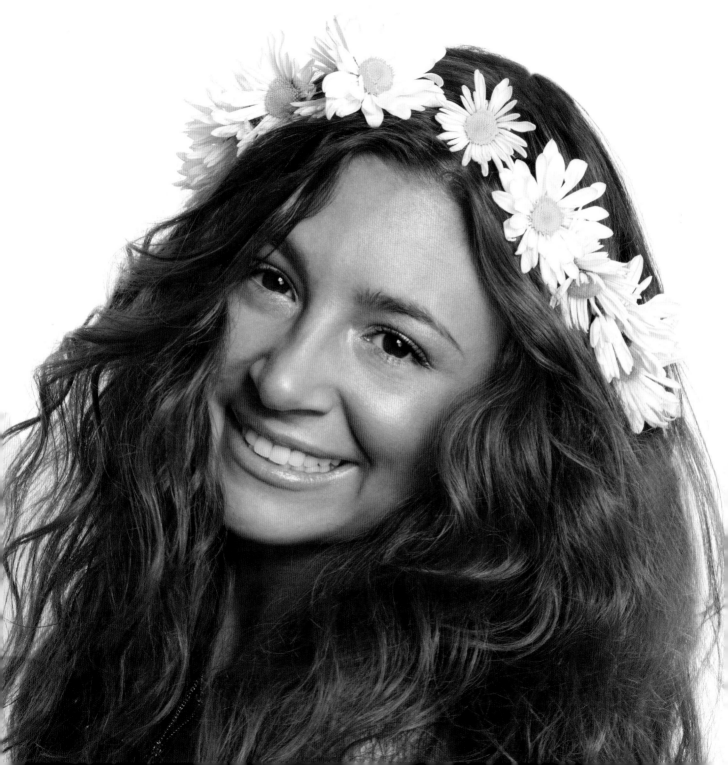

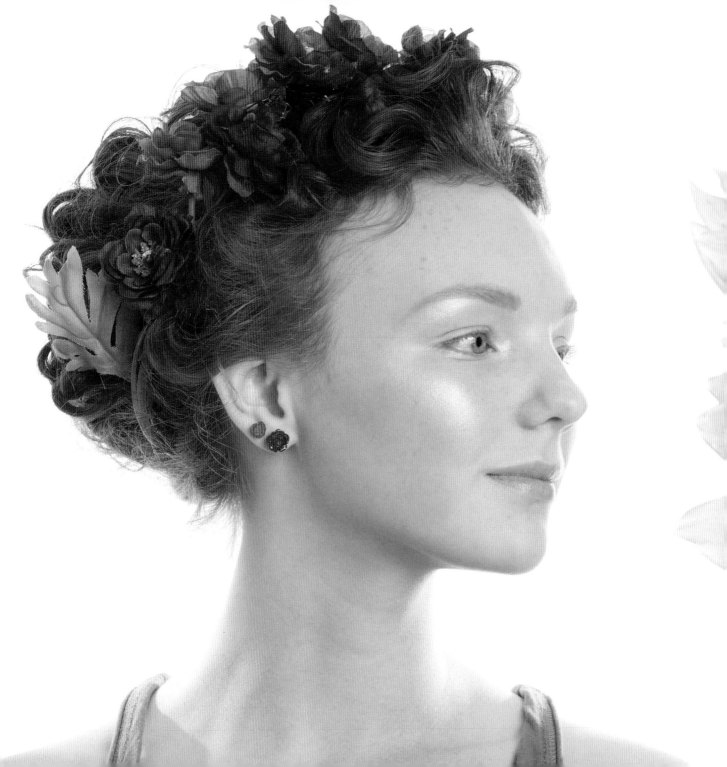

Carmindize Me!

"Carmindizing" is a cool technique I created on *What Not to Wear* to help bring light to your face in order to illuminate your natural beauty. Actually, while we're at it, think of the verb "to Carmindize" as a technique that can be applied to every aspect of your life: It's really a way to bring light, love, and radiance to everything! Here's how to Carmindize your face with a pretty, glowing look that will definitely get you noticed. Sweep a shimmering cream or powder highlighter on three key places on the skin: Directly under your brow bones, on the inside corners of your eyes near the tear ducts, and on top of your cheekbones for an ethereal, lit-from-within complexion. The highlighter will capture light, reflecting it and making your skin look luminous. If you have fair skin, go with a pearlescent hue; for medium skin, try a sparkling champagne shade; and if you have darker skin, think a glowing sunset gold.

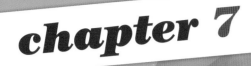

chapter 7

Kiss

AND MAKEUP

You know why I love your pretty rosebud lips so much? Because no matter what their shape or size, this expressive part of your face is all about happy smiles and the infectious laughter that teen girls are known for. Full, small, upturned, downturned, crooked, asymmetrical: Your unique lip shape is absolutely lovely in every way, so pampering your pucker is a must. Another awesome thing about lips is that from dramatic rose reds to demure peony pinks, lip color is a fun, easy way to change your look in both big and small ways!

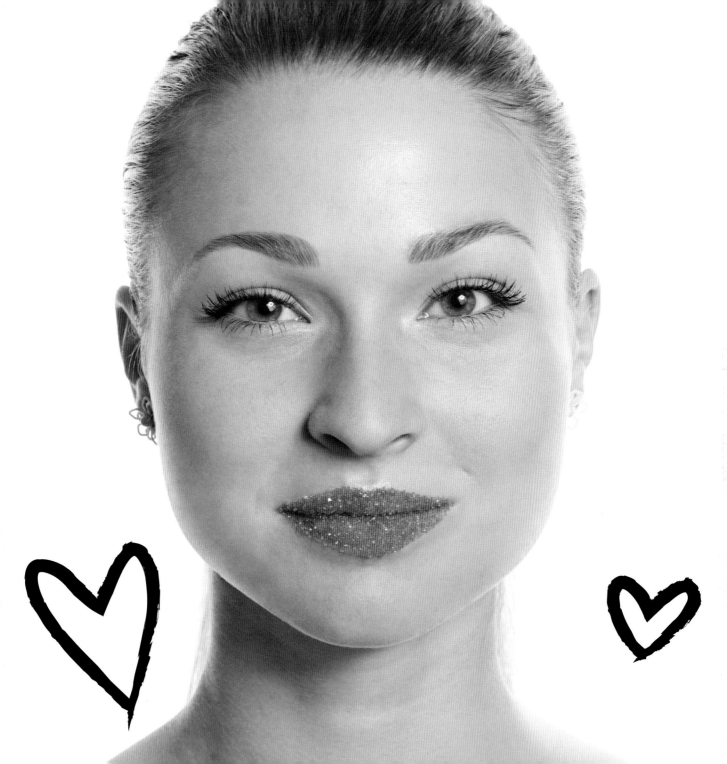

The key to getting perfectly kissable soft lips is to keep them hydrated and smooth. Nothing is worse than scaly, peeling lips that crack—which can really plague you all winter, ugh!—so it's important to take care of them. If your lips tend to get dry or chapped, here's an easy way to exfoliate them: Use a clean washcloth, a little Vaseline, and white sugar to scrub them smooth. Just apply a pinch of sugar directly on Vaseline-coated lips, grab a moist washcloth, and lightly scrub the dry skin away. Be sure to go easy and gently buff instead of aggressively wiping, as you don't want to tear the skin! When you are done, slick on a dab of all-natural lip balm to help moisturize them and keep them supple. Violà! Now you're ready to play with color.

When it comes to trends—and let's face it, they can really come and go at warp speed—lip color is the cheapest and easiest way to update your makeup wardrobe. Drugstore brands offer a wide variety of fashion-forward, of-the-moment shades that you don't need a mega allowance for. That said, when picking the right colors there are a few general rules for dealing with your own special, individual lip shape. The first one is simple: Please, *never* use colored lipliners to draw on or change your Mother Nature–approved, perfect-for-your-face lip shape. There have been fads in the past where girls and grown women alike have been known to use lip pencils to "color outside the lines" to

> Lip color is the cheapest and easiest way to update your makeup wardrobe.

make their lips look bigger, and honestly, they were not fooling anyone! Naturally plump lips are gorgeous, no question, but bigger isn't always better. Thinner, baby-doll-like lips are totally adorable and beautiful in their own right. So repeat after me: I will not color outside the lines. I will respect and celebrate my smile by enhancing it with the right lippie tip for me!

COLOR THEORY

Anyway, back to those color rules. Keep in mind these are in no way, shape, or form set in stone, and the more advanced you get with makeup, the more you'll probably want to branch out and try crazy-fun new colors like neon hues or sparkly finishes. But when you're just getting started, here are some tried-and-true rules to play it safe and go from there:

• **SMALL LIPS:** If you have one of those baby-doll pouts I was talking about earlier, slick on lighter or midtoned, neutral shades that have a bit of shimmer, which will help accentuate your dainty lips. For now, avoid super-dark, opaque shades that can make them recede. The kinds of really hard-core, intense shades that you often see in fashion mags can look a little bizarre in real life, and they require a lot of maintenance

Repeat after me: I will not color outside the lines. I will respect and celebrate my smile by enhancing it with the right lippie tip for me!

throughout the day. Can you imagine trying to reapply your lipstick on the DL in algebra class? So, if you desperately want to try a red or a deeper hue, try taking baby steps with a sheer gloss, which will give you the color pop without the mess and fuss.

- **MEDIUM-SHAPED LIPS:** The rules here are that, for the most part, there are no rules. You can certainly try most hues and textures, but because of your age (and honestly, at any age), like I've said before, less is more! There are lots of pink and berry tones that won't overpower your face, so my advice is to stick with neutral shades that let your true natural beauty shine through day-to-day and go bright and bold on special occasions. Word to the wise: If you decide to go for a major makeup color moment, keep it simple and don't add a gloss on top, which will just look too overpowering. The strong color itself will make the statement.

- **LARGER LIPS:** Be proud of that gorgeous, plump pucker! Your lips look fab in mid-tones, deep, and bright hues alike, but stay away from super shine. Thick, gloopy gloss will magnify your lips and make them look bigger. The slick look can be really overpowering on full, fabulous lips, so look for creamy, satiny finishes on your lipsticks.

The slick look can be really overpowering on full, fabulous lips, so look for creamy, satiny finishes on your lipsticks.

LIPPIE LOVE

Lip products come in an almost overwhelming variety of formulas and textures. Here are the most popular forms, why each one totally rocks, and what the heck to do with them:

• **BALMS:** Clear or tinted lip balms are the best teen choice for day-to-day protection, moisture, and sometimes a hint of color. Choose one that contains an SPF to keep your puckered pout from chapping. I really love some of the newer, super-fun tinted balms that offer a sheer blast of color. There are also balm/gloss hybrids that give the feel of a balm with a higher shine for extra kick.

Matchy-Matchy!

It's totally cool to match your lips to your nails. In fact, it looks really chic when you do! The key to rocking this look is to keep your outfit another color entirely. A few elements of the same shade can be worn in your accessories, but your actual clothing should never be overly matchy-matchy.

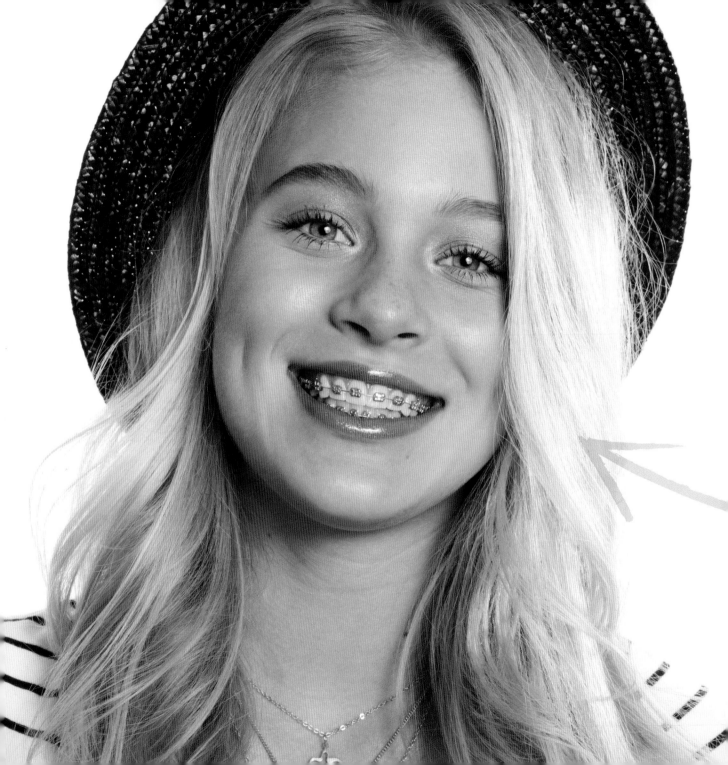

Glosses

• **GLOSSES:** I always say when in doubt . . . lip gloss! It has a magical way of brightening up your mood in a flash. Lip gloss is a really fun way to sweep on a sassy look fast, plus you can collect a different shade for every day of the week and every mood you have. Wear alone or over lipstick for a more intense look.

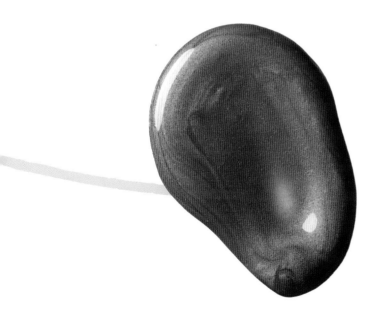

Lip Liners: To Be, or Not to Be?

My philosophy: Don't, girls, just don't. **Colored lip liners** are so dated, and you always look like you have ring around the mouth. If you really want to make your lips stand out, you can trace the outside perimeter with a Carmindizing highlighter to accentuate the shape, and then fill in the lips with whatever form of lippie you choose. That way, your lips will look glowing and fresh, without the telltale liner effect!

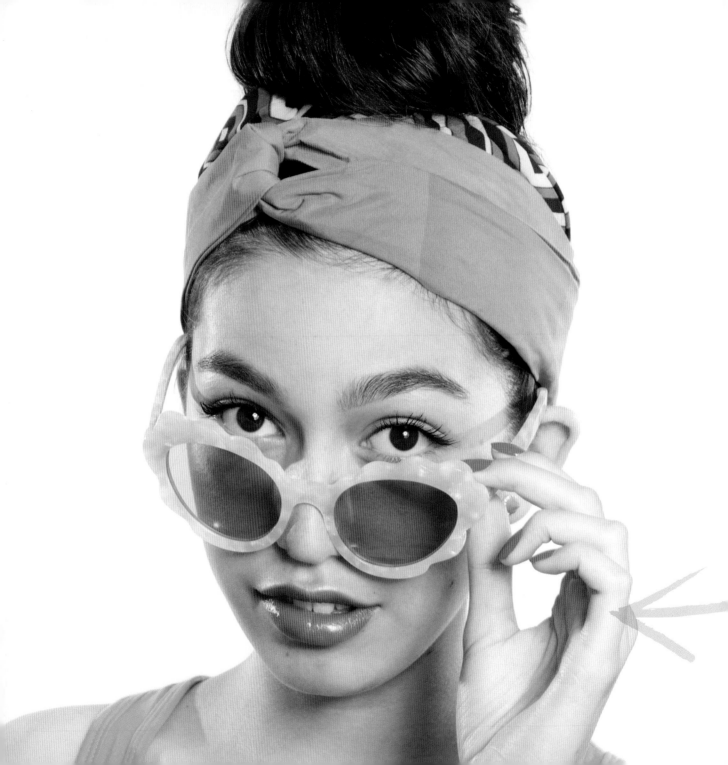

Stains

- **STAINS:** A lip stain can be a more long-wearing way to apply color to your kisser, but make sure lips are silky smooth and not chapped, because the stain can catch in dry skin and end up looking kind of gross! Use the sugar exfoliation tip I gave you earlier in this chapter for smooth lips first, then feel free to stain away. This look is great for sporty girls (you know who you are!) who are high action and don't have time to reapply.

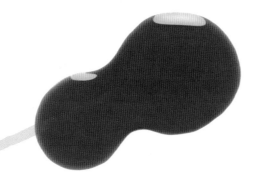

Bright Thinking

Extra-bright lip colors like hot pink, coral, orange, and red are totally modern and cool and can look incredible on teenage beauties! Here's the secret to keeping this look fully epic: Keep the rest of your makeup totally clean. Maybe you'll add a little mascara, blush, and a Carmindizing highlighter, but skip the rest so the bright lip is the star of the show and you look effortlessly fresh.

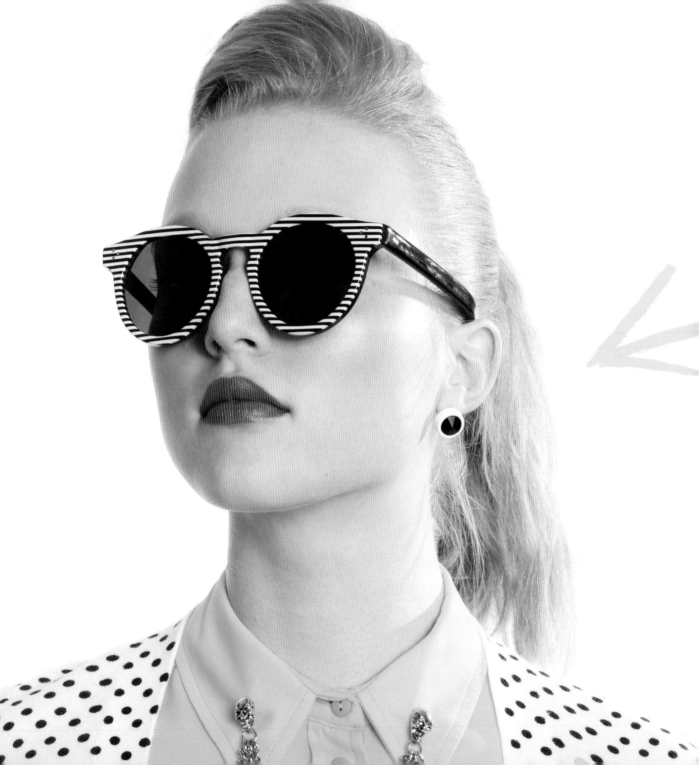

Lipsticks and Crayons

- **LIPSTICKS:** Wowza, there are literally so many lipsticks to choose from! Where do you even start? First and foremost, I say have fun playing with different shades and textures, and you might even find your own signature look. One semester you might be all about a sheer nude lip paired with a cat eye, and next it's an opaque red or orange lip paired with lots of lash. Whatever you decide, know that putting on a lipstick is a classically feminine way to make a statement. To create your own lipstick palette, buy a little plastic pill box and use a knife to cut the tops of different hues of lipstick and mush them into each sectional box. Use a retractable lip brush to apply a different one whenever the mood strikes, or even mix together a few shades to customize your own color like a true beauty pro.

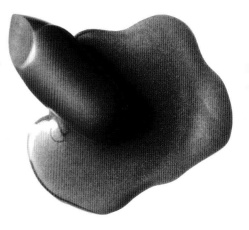

- **CRAYONS:** Lip crayons are my favorites and are a no-brainer to apply because they go on just like, well, a crayon. It's a total breeze as you use the finer tip to easily trace the lip line, turn on its side to fill in the lips, and then pop it in your purse. They come in sheer, opaque, shimmer, matte, and balm formulas, and there are just so many fun colors to play with.

RED, RED
Rose

Bright red lips never fail to make a dramatic statement and look amazing on everyone. You know what? There is a red lippie for every chickie! The key is choosing the perfect complement to your unique skin tone. If you are fair, go for reds in pinky hues like cherry or strawberry. If you have medium- or olive-toned skin, choose bright apple and fire-engine reds. For my darker-skinned maidens, think garnet and blood reds. There is also this crazy old idea that redheads should avoid red lipstick. Not true! Ginger girls can and should play with brick or tomato reds and look fabulous. If a red lipstick is too intense for you, take baby steps and try a sheer gloss, stain, or crayon that will give you a kiss of the red hue without having to fully commit to a serious red lipstick. To avoid getting red lipstick on your teeth, after applying your shade of choice, put your pointer finger in your mouth and close your lips around it. Now pull it out slowly and this will get rid of any lipstick on the inside of your lips close to your teeth. One more tip: When trying to pick your perfect shade, swipe the red lipstick, gloss, or balm on a piece of white paper instead of your hand. This way, you will more clearly be able to see what the true color is.

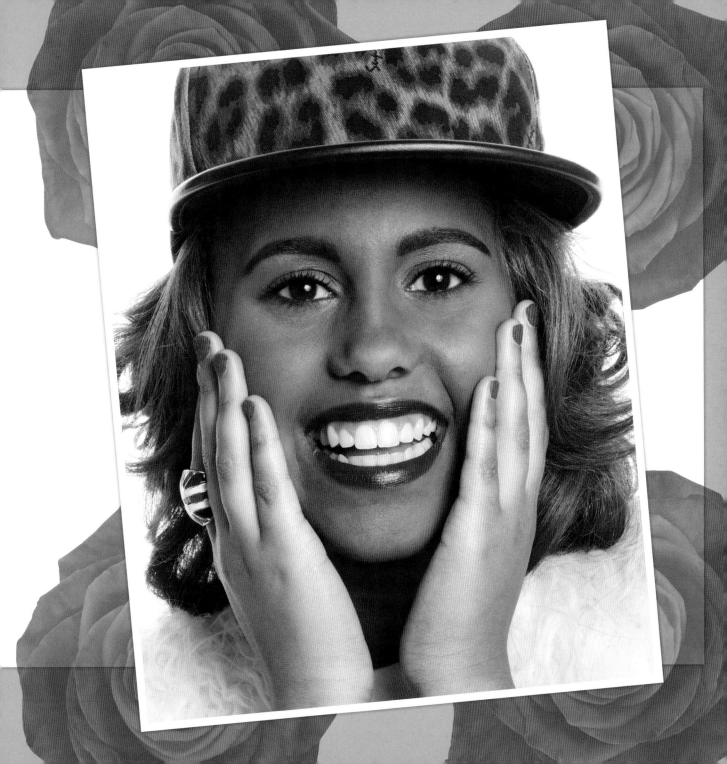

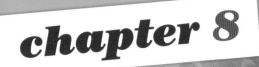

chapter 8

THE
Nasties

Okay, girls, real talk: All of us have had those OMG moments where we just want to just die of embarrassment. For me, it felt like it was all the time! When I was a teenager, I would get cold sores on my lip about twice a year. Majorly not cool. Once, in the eighth grade, I woke up with a huge one on the very day I was supposed to get up in front of the whole class to read my book report. Talk about great timing. I was so nervous that people would see it that I kept my head bowed down while

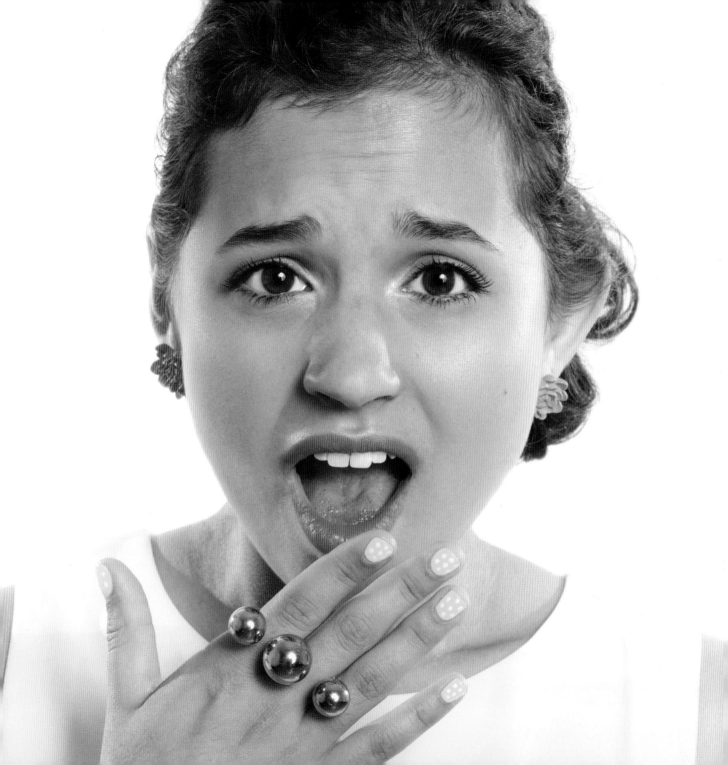

I gave my talk. Well, the worst thing that could happen actually did. Kids started calling me "herpes face"—lovely!—and boys began spreading rumors that nobody would ever want to kiss me. I was super ashamed and I showed it, which did nothing but make me an even easier target for yet more teasing.

Another time, when I was a junior in high school, I was smiling at my crush, who was sitting next to me after lunch one day. What I didn't realize is that I had a huge piece of spinach stuck in my teeth! He then asked me if I was saving it for later to snack on. Yikes!! So beyond gross, and I just wanted to crawl under my desk. I could never again bring myself to even look in his direction.

Every single one of us will experience similarly embarrassing moments or have yucky skin issues crop up unexpectedly and at the worst times possible. It's called life and we are human, and the best way to deal with these moments is to have solid self-esteem and, most of all, a great sense of humor. Laughing at yourself and giving your ego a break is the best way to downplay a potentially embarrassing, OMG situation. Whether you're suffering from an acne breakout, wart, or anything else, please, please don't waste your precious flower power on feeling ashamed. Instead, make a joke out of it; when you lighten up, others will follow your lead. If you truly don't care what others think, or at least act like you don't, then you come across as confident and powerful. Trust me! So if you get a nasty little cold sore and someone notices it, sarcastically say something like, "Oh, that's just Crusty, my pet herpe." LOL! Making others laugh at your funny way of viewing a Nasty will help take the stigma away. Plus, other kids can't really tease you if you beat them to the punch with your great attitude and ability to laugh at yourself—it's just not as fun for them if they can't get a reaction out of you! Here's an example of how this strategy worked for me: One day at school, I felt nauseous and had to leave my friends at the lunch table to go throw up. But when I got back to the table, I smiled and told them I must have gotten sick because of Pepe, my pet parasite. The laughter that followed this statement totally changed the whole mood of the situation. So, say you get a pimple in the middle of your face, and someone says something mean. The last thing you want to do is get insecure about it. Instead, say something like, "Yeah, I actually needed something to distract away from my awesomeness!" It can take time to learn this kind of confidence, but if you keep practicing, eventually it will happen. Fake it till you make it!

If you truly don't care what others think, or at least act like you don't, then you come across as confident and powerful.

HOW TO DEAL

Now that you have the tools to handle the situation on a social level, I'll give you the goods on how to diminish the physical issue in the meantime:

ZITS: If you have acne, or a breakout, or even that one Jupiter-sized zit that shows up uninvited, don't fret, my flower! Your first instinct might be to cover your whole face with heavy foundation, but that's basically just a dead giveaway that you're trying to hide something. Instead, you can simply conceal the bumps, then play the "look over here!" makeup game. Here's how: First, apply a medicated pimple cream that contains salicylic acid, sulfur, or benzoyl peroxide on the trouble spot. Next, conceal the breakout with makeup (see Chapter 2), and make sure to finish it off with a very light dusting of powder to keep it in place. (If you have a zit that's a bit scabby and dry-looking, do apply the concealer, but skip the powder step, which will just make it look more crusty.) Now, the "look over here!" makeup game is all about distracting people by choosing to play up one of your best features with a hot new makeup trend. This way you redirect the focus away from your breakout and toward your awesome hot pink lips or an electric blue cat eye everyone wants to copy. Seriously, it works! And remember: *You* may fixate on that zit and feel like everyone is staring at it, but nine times out of ten, no one notices but you!

Here's some more advice on damage control: If you feel a biggie coming on, grab an ice cube, wrap it in tissue or a thin cloth, and firmly hold it over the erupting zit to calm the swelling. A touch of lemon juice on an unbroken zit can dry it out in a flash; just don't ever do this in the daytime, as the sun can cause burning, so try it at night only. If you don't have a pimple cream handy, create an instant zit paste by mixing water with baking soda and dab it on the spot overnight to dry it up. If a cheek pimple is still visible through your blush, take a fine-tipped concealer brush and lightly dab a small mix of foundation and concealer on it. Then, using a Q-tip, pick up a little blush and face powder mixture and tap it lightly on top.

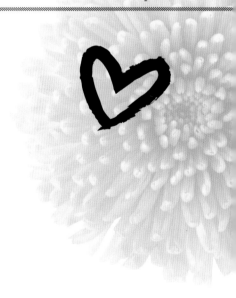

You may fixate on that zit and feel like everyone is staring at it, but nine times out of ten, no one notices but you!

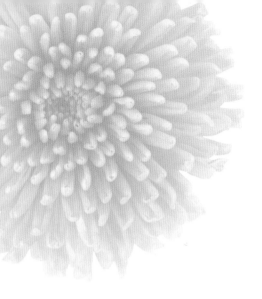

When a cold sore rears its ugly head, you must remember that they are contagious upon contact and can spread.

COLD SORES: I especially hate these Nasties because I personally have had to deal with them since I was a kid. If you're prone to them and cold sores are a major, recurring issue, you might want to ask your parents to look into getting you a prescription from your doctor or dermatologist for medicine like Valtrex so you can get a jump-start on healing the moment you feel "the tingle" that always seems to precede them. When a cold sore rears its ugly head, you must remember that they are contagious upon contact and can spread. Don't kiss anyone or share drinks or utensils, as the cold sore can transfer to others.

So, if it's too late to prevent and the sore has already formed, you can conceal it in a way that won't look crusty and also won't contaminate the rest of your makeup. (You don't want to use any of your makeup brushes because the virus is contagious; instead, use disposable Q-tips and non-latex sponges to camouflage the area.) Begin by applying a dab of cold sore cream with a Q-tip, and then squeeze a bit of foundation and/or concealer on the back of your hand. Next, take a fresh Q-tip, dip into the concealer, and lightly dab it over the sore. When you're done, take a non-latex sponge, dip it

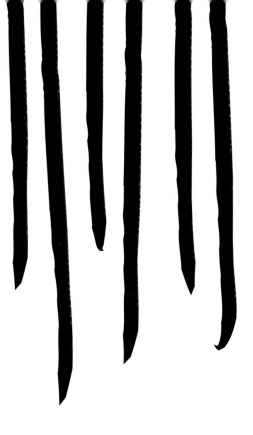

into a light, translucent powder, and gently press it on top of the sore to set the makeup. Another way to conceal the issue is to try one of those cold sore concealing patches and apply it directly over the sore on clean skin. Once it adheres, you can then blend on the foundation, concealer, or powder in the same sterile way I described directly on top of the patch and the sore will be protected underneath. (The patches easily peel off when you get home and you can reapply your medicine then.) And make sure not to pick or touch the sore! One last thing: If the sore is around the lips, don't use a shiny lip gloss or bold lip color, as this will just draw the eye to the area where the cold sore is. Instead choose a neutral, natural-looking pink or rose shade in the form of a tinted lip balm or sheer lipstick, and again, be sure to apply it using a disposable Q-tip so you don't contaminate your lip products.

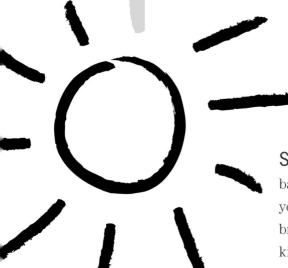

There's certainly nothing cute about bright red skin, plus burns can be painful and cause all kinds of nasty skin conditions later in life.

SUNBURNS: You guys know this already, but basically, sunburns are the absolute worst beauty sin you can commit! There's certainly nothing cute about bright red skin, plus burns can be painful and cause all kinds of nasty skin conditions later in life. Trust me, avoid them at all cost! If you do accidently get sunburned, then there are a few easy ways to ease the pain: The first quick fix is to take an aspirin or ibuprofen to reduce pain and inflammation. To sooth crispy, fried skin, run a cold bath, add a cup of good old-fashioned oatmeal or baking soda, and then soak your bod for about twenty minutes. When you emerge, let yourself air dry, because drying off with a towel might irritate the sensitive skin. Slather yourself in an aloe vera–based moisturizer the moment you're dry in order to both moisturize your parched skin and to start the healing process at the same time. To hide a burn, use a non-latex sponge and "stipple" (a quick patting motion) liquid foundation gently over the reddened area, then finish with a yellow-tinted powder that will counteract any redness that might show through.

PERIODS: That dreaded time of the month sometimes arrives unexpectedly and can totally ruin your day, especially if you are wearing light-colored clothing. Don't let it! Get to know your menstruation schedule by downloading a period planner off the Internet or as a phone app, and always be prepared. If you know you are getting close, opt to wear darker-colored clothing that week, and always carry what I like to call an "Aunt Flo Kit" in your purse or backpack. Here's how to make one: Find or make a small zippered pouch, and stock it with all of your must-have precautionary items so you can be in control of your flow, on the go.

THE AUNT FLO KIT: A few tampons and pads; Midol (in case of cramping); dandelion root supplements (for bloating); and a small piece of dark chocolate (to satisfy cravings and give you a jolt of good-for-you antioxidants). Breakouts and cold sores also tend to crop up during your period (I know, jeez!), so throw in a small tube of spot treatment cream, a concealer, and a cold sore lip balm. Monthly mishaps beware, now you are prepared!

Get to know your menstruation schedule by downloading a period planner off the Internet or as a phone app, and always be prepared.

Just keep in mind that the rotten times don't last, and everything will be okay in the end.

BOOGIES: A "bat in the cave" can be a total OMG moment, so it helps to always have a small pocket mirror and a purse-sized pack of Q-tips handy so you can do a tunnel check throughout the day. Again, if you get busted with a boogie, make a funny joke out of it; that's the best way to deflect a potential "wanna crawl into the ground" moment.

BODY ODOR: It's super easy to avoid embarrassing body odor by swiping on a fresh-smelling deodorant as soon as you get out of the shower each and every day. Keep a mini-sized travel one in your backpack or purse if you have to shower again in gym class or after any sweat-inducing activities you may be involved in. A scented body spray and breath mints will also keep you sweetly scented from head to toe.

PUFFY, CRIED-OUT EYES: Girls, even the most positive petunias out there have good times and bad. Just keep in mind that the rotten times don't last, and everything will be okay in the end. And if it's not . . . it's not the end. Things will get better. That said, a heavy-duty cry fest (or just a night spent tossing and turning) can leave your eyes swollen and puffy—*so* not a good look! In order to de-puff crybaby eyes, here are a few

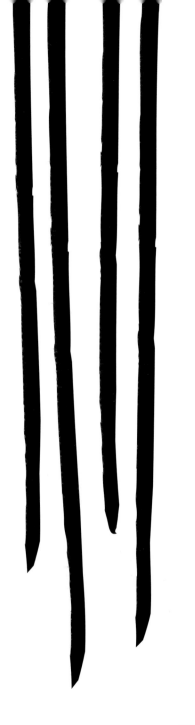

easy, quick-fix tips to help erase any signs of sadness: Pop two wet, metal spoons in the freezer. When they're good and chilled, gently hold them over swollen eyes to ease the swelling. Or, steep a couple of black tea bags (the kind that contains caffeine), stick them in the fridge until they're ice-cold, and hold them under your eyes to tighten and soothe the area. One more: A tried-and-true spa favorite is to slice cold cucumbers, then press the thin veggie discs over the eyes to help ease the baggage.

BIKINI LINE BUMPS: If you're headed to the beach and shaving has left you with a visible bikini rash, use a spray foundation to spritz coverage over the rash. (Lots of drugstore makeup brands make these now.) Use a non-latex sponge to dab over the spray, blending it into the skin. Violà, erased!

BRUISES: To cover up purplish, unsightly bruises, conceal those bad boys by using a simple layering technique. First, dab a slightly orange-tinted thick concealer over the bruise, which will counteract the purple hue. Next, spritz spray foundation (one that matches your skin tone) over the area. Last, lightly dust a translucent powder over the top of the bruise to set the makeup so that it will stay in place.

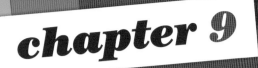

chapter 9

LET'S GET
Interactive

Whether it's through my website or other forms of social media like Facebook, Twitter, and Instagram, girls come to me all the time with questions and concerns about beauty. These cyber portholes present amazing opportunities for me to help navigate young women through the confusing world of beauty products, conflicting information, weird YouTube videos, and crazy makeup trends that seem to change with the wind.

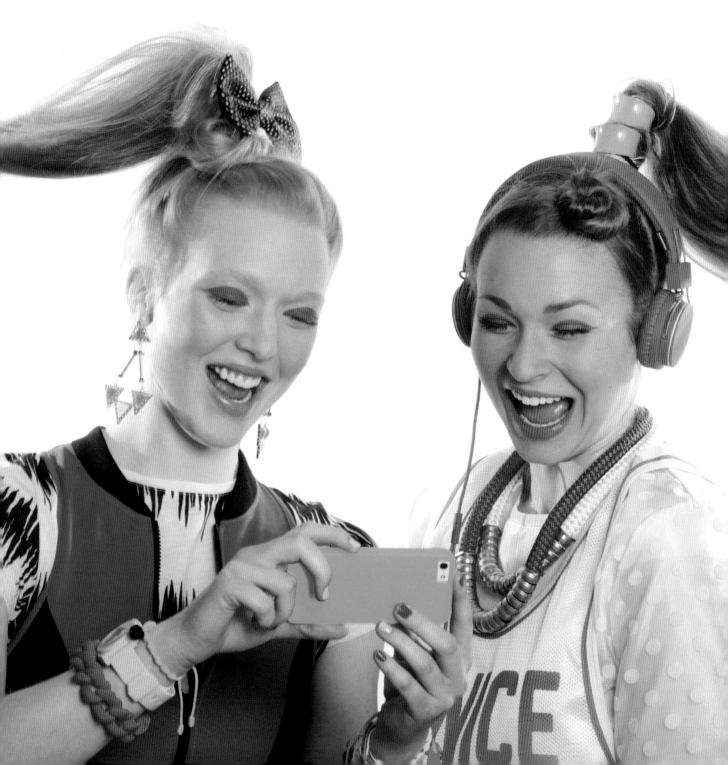

When in doubt, it's totally helpful to consult a beauty expert (like me) or a beauty blogger who you trust and whose style you love so you can learn the insider tips and tricks that will work best for you. The Internet is also a great place to find all kinds of makeup deals, specialty beauty products from around the globe, and new makeup styles you may want to try. Smartphones can also be majorly fun tools when it comes time to trying cool, trendy makeup looks, and you can bring your friends in on the action too. If you want to try a new, hot makeup trend for a special event, use your smartphone to snap selfies of you wearing different looks, then share them with your friends on Instagram. You can ask them to vote on which ones they like the best. Then rock the winning look at a school dance or a birthday party. You can also use Pinterest to create your own beauty boards that you can reference in the future whenever you need that extra jolt of inspiration.

That said, and please don't take this as a lecture—I know you get enough of that at home and at school!—often, when I engage with girls on social media, I can't help but notice that many profile pictures can be, well, *inappropriate*. I really can't stress it enough: When it's time to create your profile and your profile pictures, it's best to take your time, step back a minute, and think about what kind of image you really want to project to the world. Remember that once it's out there in the Internet ether, it's hard to take it back, so always walk on the side of caution. Keep things humble and subtle, and don't throw it all out there at once. Think of it this way: By not oversharing, you get to keep up an element of mystery, which is what keeps you intriguing to your friends. The worst mistake I see time and time again is being overly sexy. That is just going to get you the wrong type of attention! You don't have to try so hard. Your outward appearance should reflect your inner love and light. Show off your personal style with a fun, natural-looking picture—whether you're smiling, serious, outrageous, or classic, whatever your personality might be—and stay true to who you are. The "5-Minute Face for Teens" (Chapter 4) is the perfect fast and easy look to rock for your profile pic. It's basically a polished version of your natural beauty. The most important thing to think about is how you want to present yourself not only visually but also personally.

Think of it this way: By not oversharing, you get to keep up an element of **mystery,** which is what keeps you intriguing to your friends.

There are so many lies and untruths online, so being your authentic self and not pretending to be something you're not is definitely the better way to go.

Another thing I'd like you to keep in mind is that there have been studies that indicate long periods of time spent online can sometimes lead to low self-esteem in teenage girls. Why? I think it's because you may be focusing on the wrong types of images. Perfectly retouched images of models and celebs online can make you play that icky "compare and despair" game where there are no winners. Remember what a unique, special flower you are, and showcase yourself with pride. If anyone ever makes a negative comment about you online, simply blow it off! By letting lame comments

The Digital "Diet"

It is important to take the time to step away from social media and really connect—face-to-face—with the people you care about on a daily basis. Smartphones and all other types of technology are awesome, but when you are so busy filming, photographing, or texting every single amazing moment, chances are you might be completely missing the experience because you are not being present and grounded in that moment. Magical memories are just as important as digital ones, so it's cool to try to keep a balance. Weirdly, spending so much time on social media can sometimes leave you feeling disconnected from friends and family, and your real-time relationships can suffer. Make sure you step away from the digital devices at times, build stronger relationships, and make *real-life* face time a priority.

affect you, you're just playing into their game. Retaliating is a waste of your beautiful energy and does not serve you at all. What *does* serve you? Letting go of negativity, moving forward with joy and confidence, and loving your unique natural beauty is all you need to focus on in order to continue to bloom into the amazing flower you are.

When you shine from within and share that glow online and on social media, the positive and beautiful vibes that radiate from you will attract all kinds of like-minded people. It's the simple law of attraction: What you put out, you get back. So, ladies, can you please make a commitment to both of us? Let's agree to give out positivity, truth, humbleness, modesty, creativity, intelligence, and love, and that is what we will get back in return.

How to Take an Awesome Profile Pic

Taking an awesome profile pic to share with your online universe is all about lighting and capturing the right angles. The no-fail way to always look your best is to never face straight toward the camera. If you turn a bit sideways—almost three-quarters—and tilt your head slightly upward or downward (practice which looks best), and hold your arm slightly away from your body, you will nail it! Try to always use a flash because it's more flattering, and don't take pictures with direct overhead sunlight or indoor florescent lighting. This will just cause shadows that aren't even there. For great pose inspiration, you can always check out pics of celebs on the red carpet. They have practiced a lot and know exactly which angles work, so try mimicking their stances.

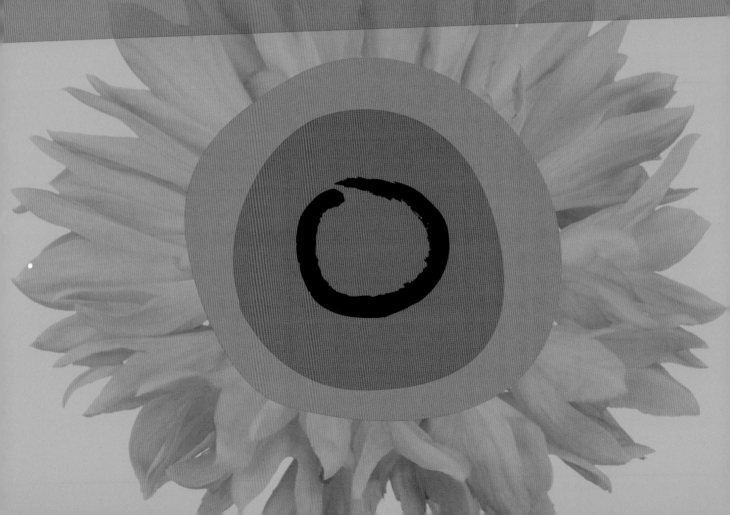

chapter 10

WHAT TO WEAR

ON YOUR *Face*

Special occasions in your budding social life set the stage to experiment with fun new makeup looks that can help you define your personality and enhance your inner flower power. From making a good impression on your first day of school to primping yourself pretty for the big "P" (prom!), your makeup can say as much about you as what clothes you choose to wear. The key is to full-on *own your look* and rock it with the kind of fun-loving confidence that creates a wave of positivity all around you. So if your style is "geek chic" or "goth goddess," be sure to celebrate, have a good time, and hey, laugh a little!

CLASS PHOTO

Ah, those infamous school pictures! You can't possibly imagine this right now, but you will probably be looking back at these pics for the rest of your life. Don't do what most of us did in the past (guilty!) and go for a super-trendy look of the moment, as it will be out of style by next year, let alone in a few decades from now. Save yourself the embarrassment. Choose to wear something timeless, go for a clean makeup look to enhance your natural beauty, and keep your hair simple so you can look back with pride. And one more thing: Smile! No sulky teen angst photos, you hear me, girls? You will thank me later.

get the look

After prepping your face, draw espresso brown eyeliner on the upper lash lines, and apply black mascara on the top lashes only. Swirl pink cream or powder blush onto the apples of your cheeks. Last, slick on a rose-tinted lip balm.

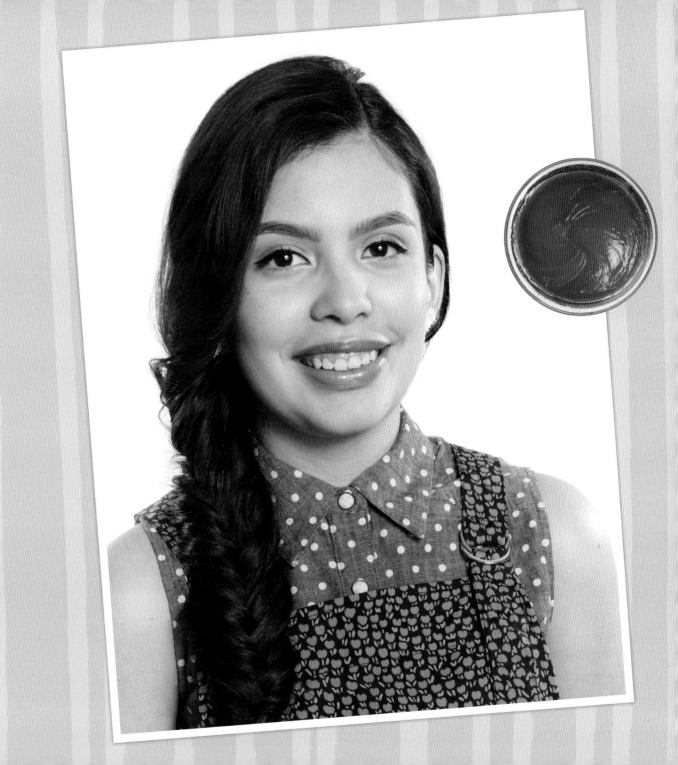

FIRST DAY OF SCHOOL

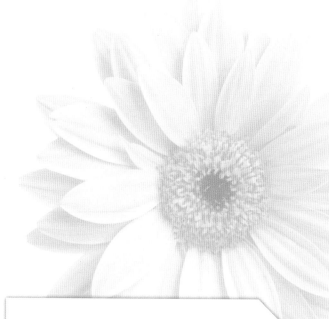

As far as I'm concerned, I think the first day of school is as much fun as prom! It's that one special day to set the tone of who you are going to be for the rest of the year. It's all about making first impressions, so you will most definitely want to start the year off showing everyone how awesome you are. Spend the last few weeks of summer creating a Pinterest board of what inspires you, and you'll start to get a feel for the kind of look you want to project in the new school year. Put together about a week's worth of looks to get the ball rolling for back-to-school, and play with makeup ahead of time so you will feel mega confident unveiling your epic look.

This is really the time to express yourself, so if you are a rock chick, a retro babe, a conservative cutie, or a glamour girl, now is your time to shine.

get the look

For this rockin' look, start by swirling on pink blush. Line the upper and lower water lines of your eyes with a black eyeliner pencil, and apply black mascara. Fill in lips using a deep plum lip crayon. Choose a dark nail color to add a bit of edge to the finished look.

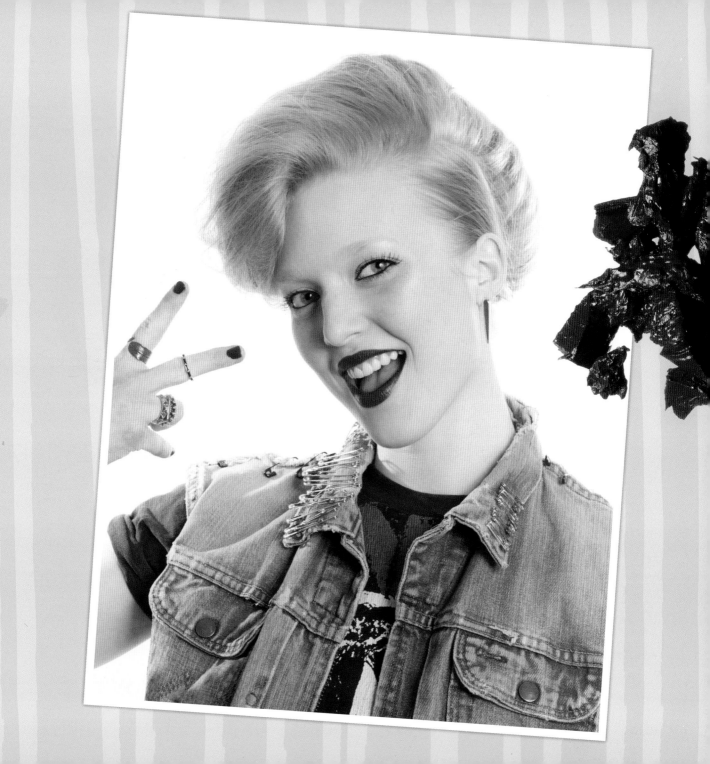

SWEET SIXTEEN

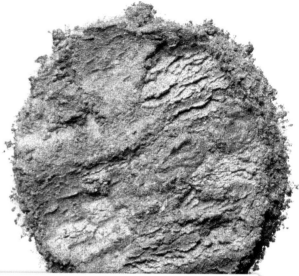

You're only sixteen once, so think fun, festive, and oh-so-sweet! This is your day to play, so try a metallic twist and a little face flair for an extra party-ready look. Choose *one* feature (like the tops of your cheeks) to enhance with this trendy makeup look, and use glitter, bindis, face decals, or an easily removable temporary tattoo to decorate your face.

get the look

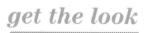

After prepping, swirl on a warm, bronzy blush. Sweep a silver metallic eye shadow across the upper lids, and add a few false lashes to the outer corners of your lash line. Lightly line the upper lash line with black liquid liner in order to hide the seam of the false lashes. Sweep black mascara on upper lashes only, and slick on a bronzy lip gloss. Finally, place a few crystal face stickers on the side of your face right above your cheekbone. Create a simple little sun pattern like this one by applying a larger crystal in the center, then add five smaller ones around it. Or get really creative with your own crazy bling design.

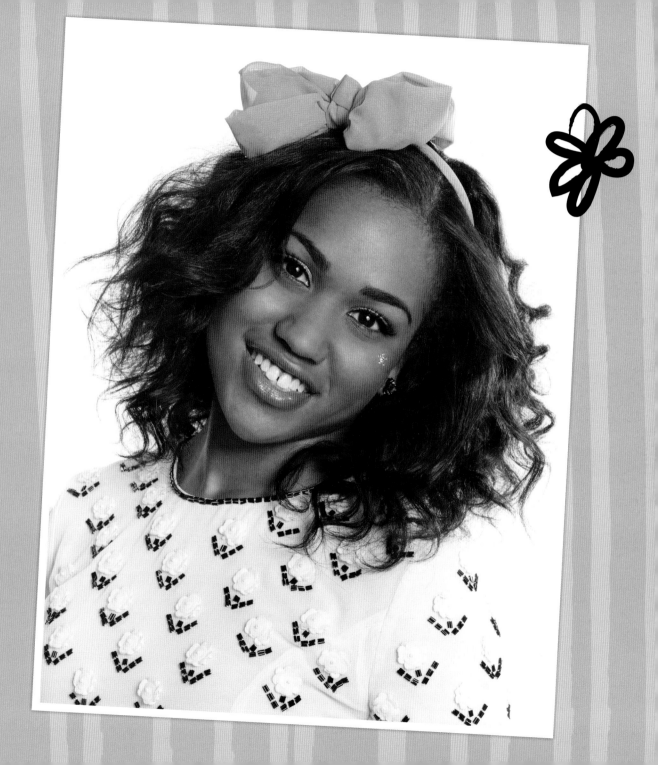

QUINCEAÑERA

Latina lovelies celebrate a year earlier than the traditional Sweet Sixteen. The word "Quinceañera" loosely translates to the celebration of a girl's fifteenth birthday. This event represents her transition from childhood into womanhood, not unlike a Bat Mitzvah for younger Jewish girls. The Quinceañera is treated almost like a debutante's ball, so chances are it's yummily over-the-top with sparkling crowns, fluffy Cinderella-style dresses, and big production-style dance routines. You can definitely push your makeup boundaries a little bit and play with fun-colored hairpieces for a little extra glitz on this glamorous birthday.

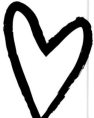

get the look

Use a variety of metallic hues to play up your eyes. First, sweep gold eye shadow across the lids from the lash line to the crease. Next, use a smaller brush to add a dot of silver metallic shadow on the center of each of your the lids. Blend on a bronze shimmer eye shadow in the crease, at the outer corner of the lids and under lower lash lines. Line the upper lash lines with black eyeliner, and apply black mascara on the tops and bottoms of the lashes. Swirl on a bronzey, berry-hued blush and choose a super shiny lip gloss in a similar shade to play up the lips. Last, clip in a fun blue hairpiece for a streak of chic and you are ready to dance the night away.

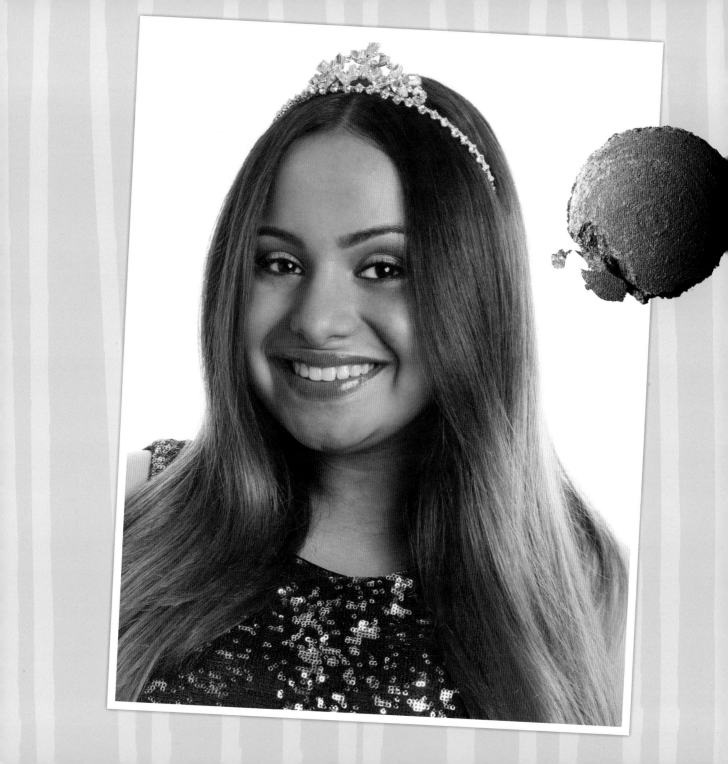

FIRST DATE

So he *finally* asked (or maybe you did!), and you and your crush are going on your first date ever. OMG, what to wear? Well, it's simple: When it comes to makeup, less, my darlings, is much more. After all, he wants to hang out because he likes you for *you*—not a fake, made-up version of you—so trust me, be true to yourself and keep it light. If you want to play up one feature, then always focus on the eyes for a flirty, come-hither look. And while a soft-colored eye shadow can help create some drama, it's best to stick to either nothing on the lips or a sheer tinted lip balm at most. Guys definitely don't want to kiss a goopy bright mouth at the end of the night because they think it will get all over them. Pick a yummy-flavored, natural-looking tinted lip balm, so if he does go in for a good-night kiss, your lips will taste delicious!

get the look

Line the upper and lower lash lines with a black eyeliner pencil, lightly smudging it by going back over your lines with a Q-tip or an angle brush. From where you applied the liner to the crease of your lids, sweep on a pale, quartz-purple shadow, then blend it into the Carmindizing highlight under your brows. Apply black mascara on the top and bottom lashes. Swirl on a romantic pink blush, then apply a natural pink lip tint in a flavor he might like. Here's a hot tip on perfume for all my fragrance-loving flowers out there: To avoid overdoing it, spritz your favorite scent in one squirt above your head, then let it lightly shower down on you so you emit a subtle scent and not a heavy, overpowering dose of perfume.

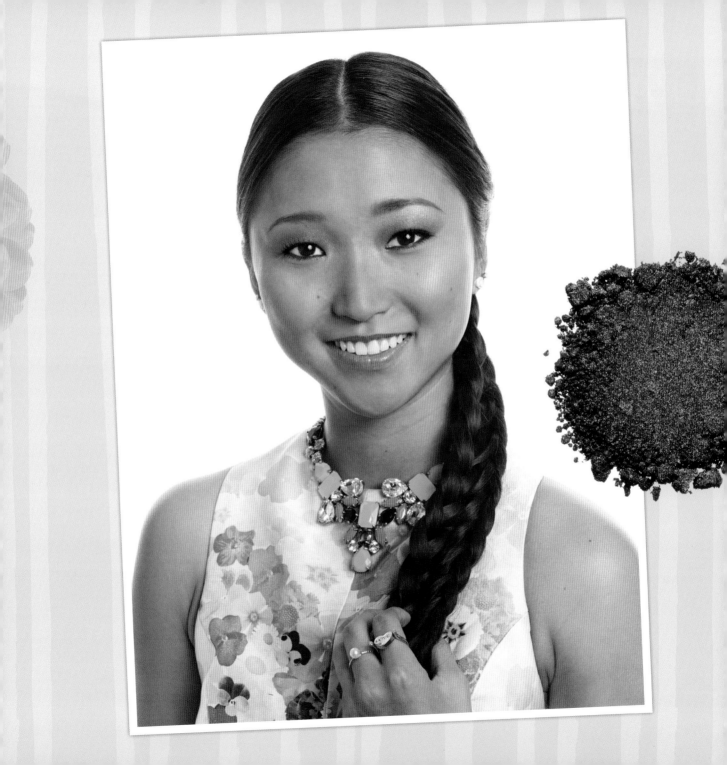

PARTY TIME

So you've just been invited to an awesome party and you really want to make a major splash. What should you do? Now is the time to simply *go for it* and try the totally trendy looks you've always wanted to experiment with. After all, a party is the perfect time to push the envelope! If it's a smoky eye you have been dying to try or the major red-lipped look of the moment, don't be afraid to try something new and have a blast doing it. I always like to apply a new look the night before the event, and then take a selfie snapshot to see if it works in photos. If it looks fierce, then by all means do it!

get the look

Choose a sparkling, metallic eye shadow like copper, and sweep it across your lids from the lash line to the crease. Next, apply black pencil eyeliner along the upper and lower lash lines and on the inside water line for added drama. Sweep on black mascara on the top and bottom lashes, then swirl on a bit of peachy-pink blush. Slick on a bright and bold red lip gloss, then walk into that party like you own the place!

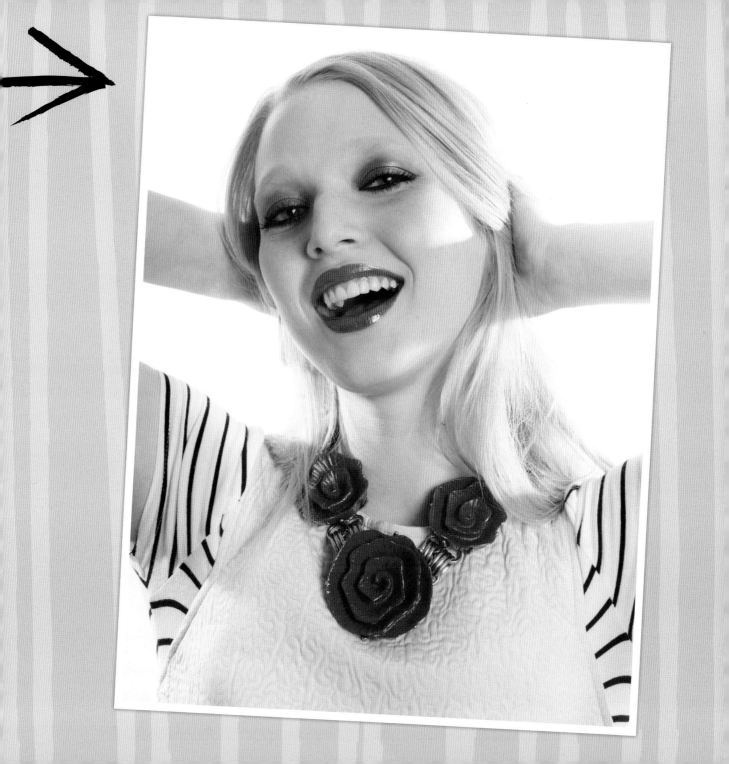

PROM

Prom is like the Academy Awards of high school, so wearing the right makeup style feels mega important! There are so many different styles and looks you can choose from for the biggest night of the year—and you can even create one of your own—but a classic, timeless look for prom has always been that of the romantic, soft goddess. Any girl can pull this off and look beyond beautiful doing so. To achieve this perfect prom style, you want to think pink, floral, and ethereal like the Greek and Roman mythological creatures you might be studying. The key to this look is blending on iridescent shimmer that will give you a goddess-y glow like no other.

get the look

Use an iridescent cream shimmer highlighter to Carmindize your face under the eyebrows on the brow bone, on the inside corners of the eyes, and on top of the cheekbones. (Bonus tip: If your arms are exposed, sweep any extra down your arms!) Next, use a shadow brush to apply a silvery-mauve pearl eye shadow across your eyelids from the lash lines to the creases, and very lightly apply extra under your lower lash lines. Use black mascara on the top and bottom lashes. Use a petal pink blush on the apples of the cheeks, and blend it back into the hairline. Finish the look with a sweep of matching petal pink lip gloss or lipstick that just whispers, "Bow down to this goddess!"

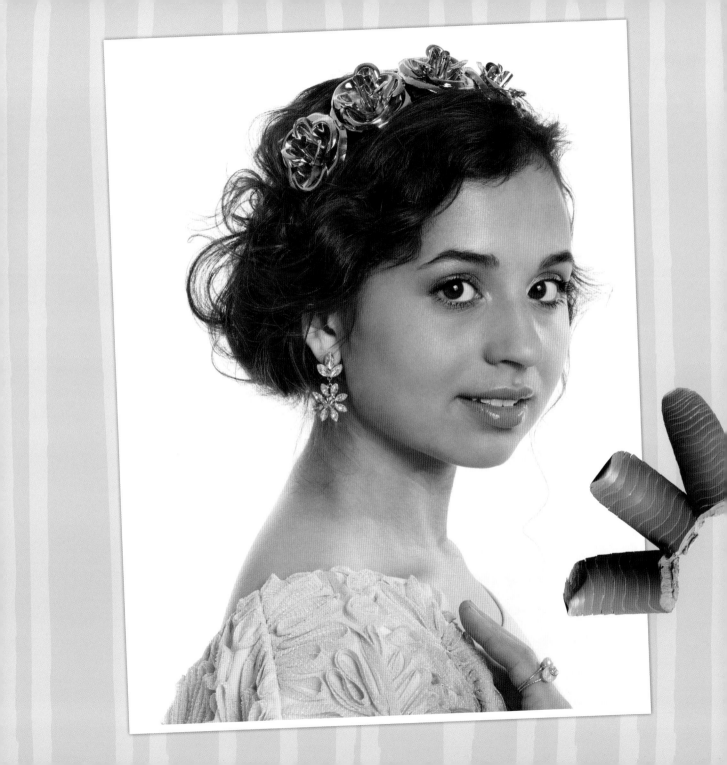

ATHLETICS

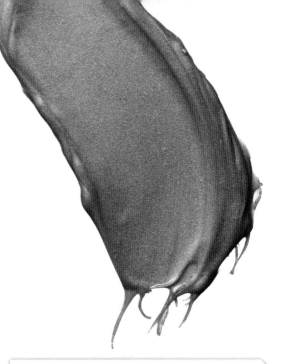

Sporty Spice girls don't have to go makeup-free just because they tend to sweat it out a bit more than their nonathletic sisters. The "5-Minute Face for Teens" is exactly the way to go when playing sports, running track, or working out so you can look polished to perfection without feeling like you have any makeup on at all. Always keep a handy pack of blotting sheets, mattifying lotion or gel, waterproof mascara, and a good SPF in your purse or backpack to stay shine-free and protected while outdoors.

get the look

Apply a waterproof mascara on the upper lashes only, and swirl on a bit of gel blush, which will last longer than cream or powder when you're sweating. Finish the look with a pretty light pink lip gloss, or try a lip stain, which will have staying power through your sweat session.

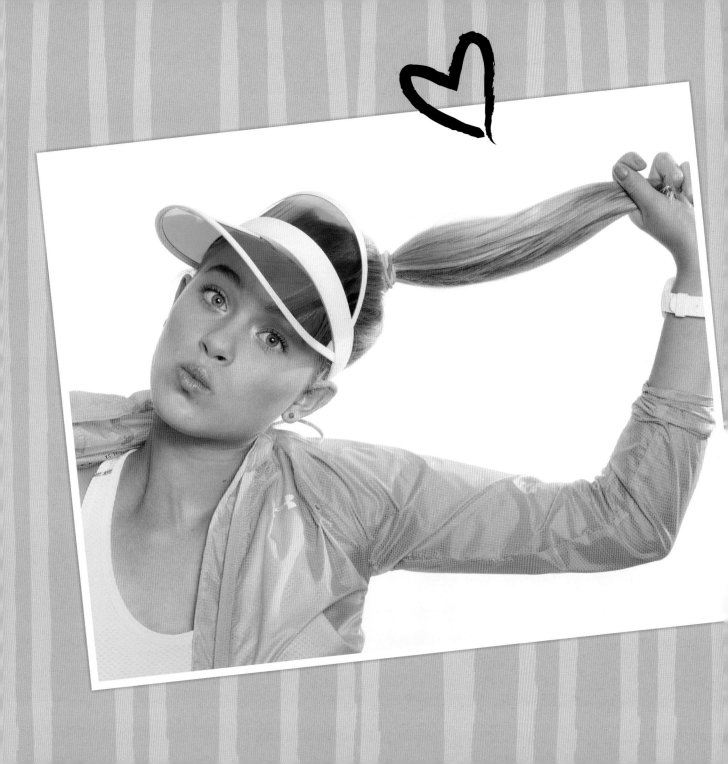

HONORS BANQUET

Okay, smarty-pants, it's time to be honored for your brains! Since you're so clever, the only unanswered question is what to wear on your face. It's an easy one: Making a statement with a strong mouth shows unparalleled confidence and lets people know just how sharp, sophisticated, and on top of your game you are. Go for a bold, sheer lippie, and you'll be a winner every time. Even presidents have focus groups that tell them wearing bold colors like red raise their approval ratings, so pay attention and be a power player.

get the look

Sweep a Bambi brown eye shadow across your lids from the lash line to the crease. Apply black mascara on the top lashes only, and swirl on a bit of pink blush to the apples of your cheeks. Make your mouth stand out with a sheer, power red lipstick so if you give a speech, everyone will be hanging on to your every word. (They'll also be wondering where you got the great lip color!)

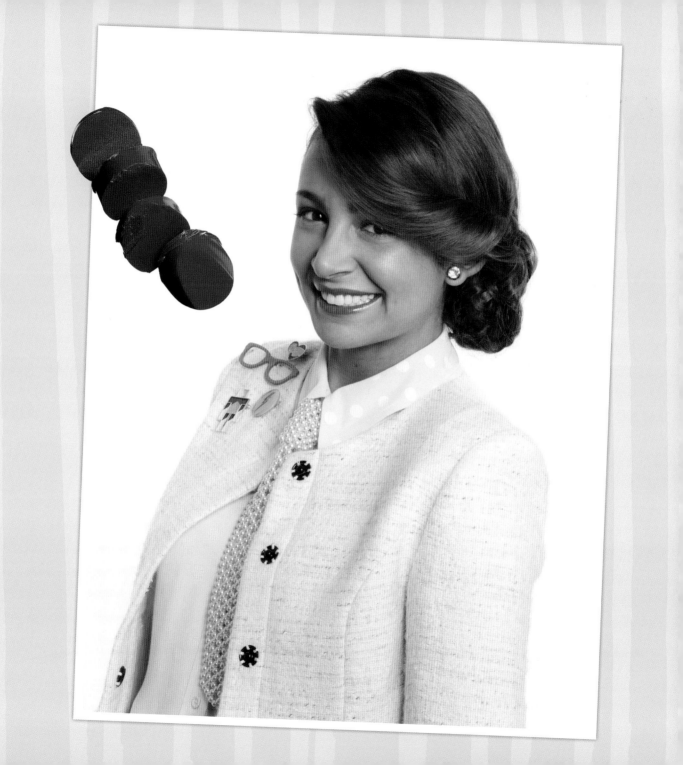

COLLEGE INTERVIEW

Going to a college interview can be exciting and even a bit scary at the same time, but showing people you have what it takes to achieve should be apparent on the outside as well as the inside. Now is the time to tone down any over-the-top personal style you have and be a little more conservative in your approach. That doesn't mean that you completely let go of certain elements of your signature style, but it is best to keep it light and focus on one area at a time. The eyes are your best bet! When you're getting ready for an interview, use my "opposites attract" technique of using eyeliner that's the opposite hue of your iris in order to leave a lasting good impression.

get the look

Start by swirling on a natural coral blush to the apples of your cheeks. Line the upper lash line with eyeliner in a contrasting hue. If your eyes are brown, try sapphire blue; if they're green, go for amethyst; if they're blue, choose burgundy brown; and if they are hazel, apply forest green. Polish off the look with a little black mascara and a natural-looking sheer coral lip gloss. This style will project an image that says, "I am an achiever and a total success." Here's to your future, my blooming beauty!

No matter what the occasion, always remember this: Each and every flower is unique, special, and, most of all, beautiful!

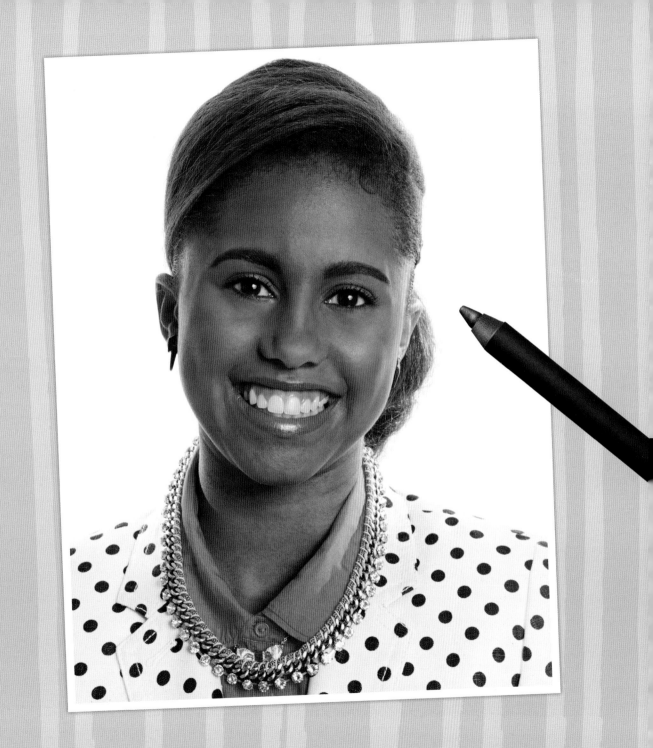

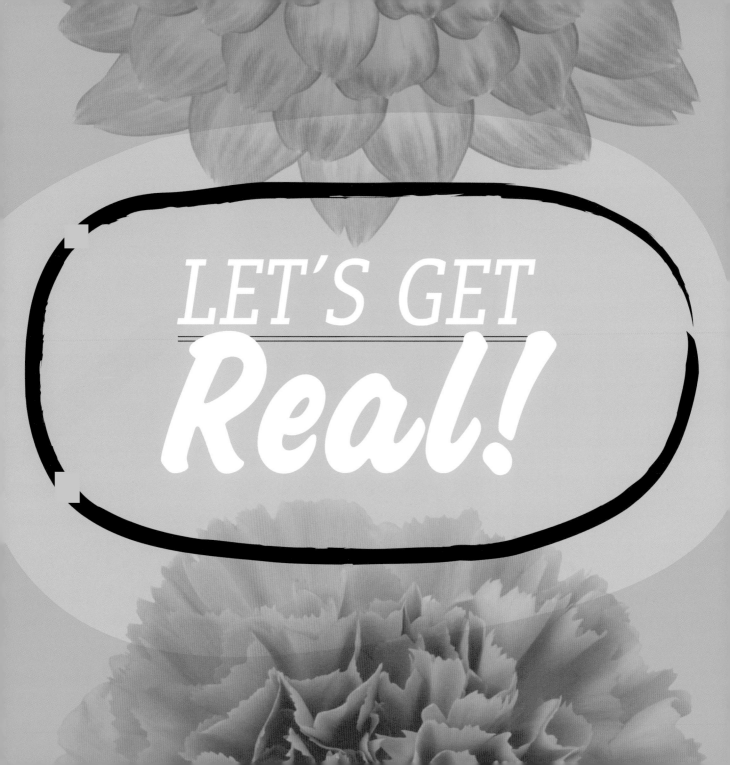

When I began this project, I was already majorly inspired by teen girls. But after meeting each of the ladies featured in these pages, I was positively blown away! These girls truly exemplify the Bloom spirit— they are confident, fun-loving, wicked smart, and most of all, beautiful both inside and out. We had a blast playing with various totally age-appropriate makeup looks that prove small tweaks can make big impacts. Because they're all so unique, these pretty flowers truly represent the idea of different kinds of beauty, just like all of you.

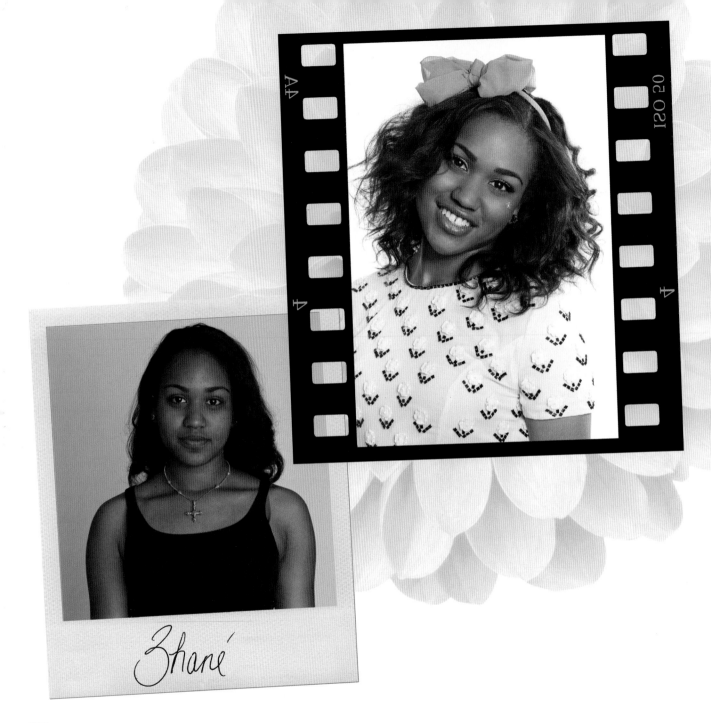

Zhané

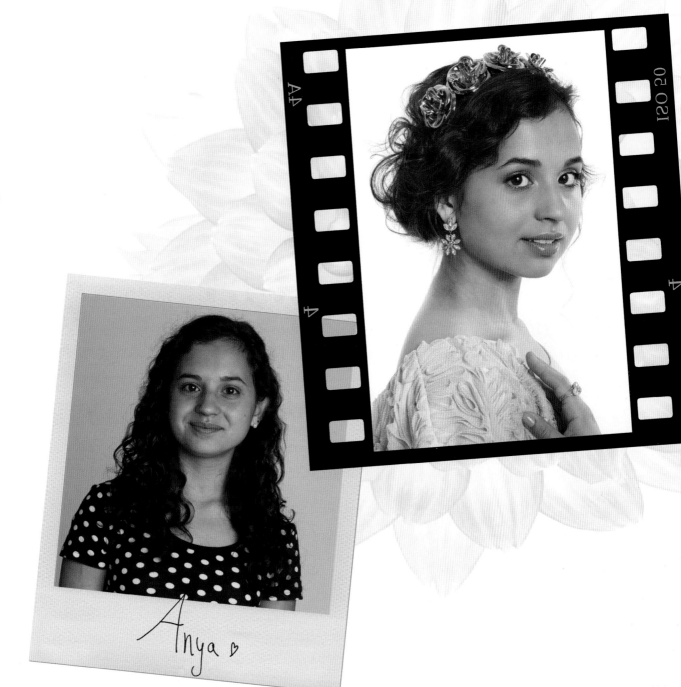

Anya ♡

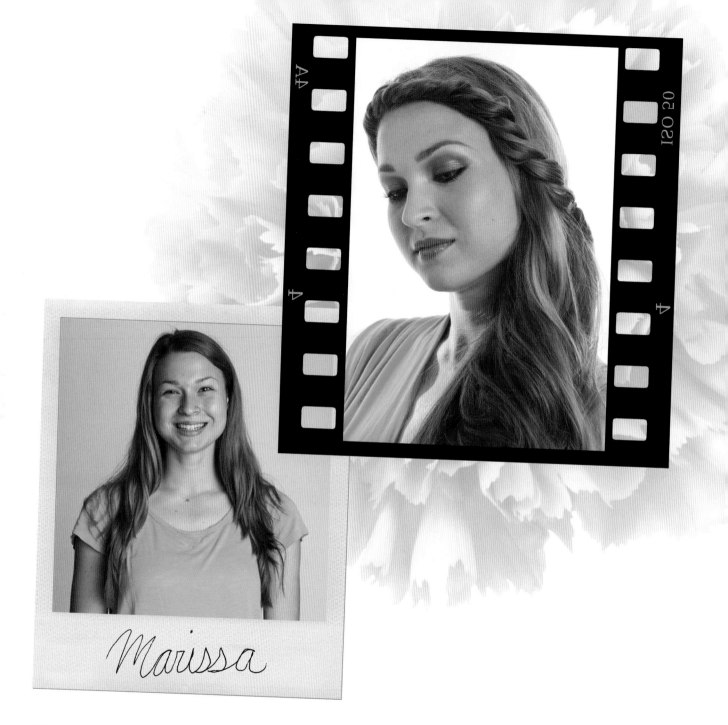

Marissa

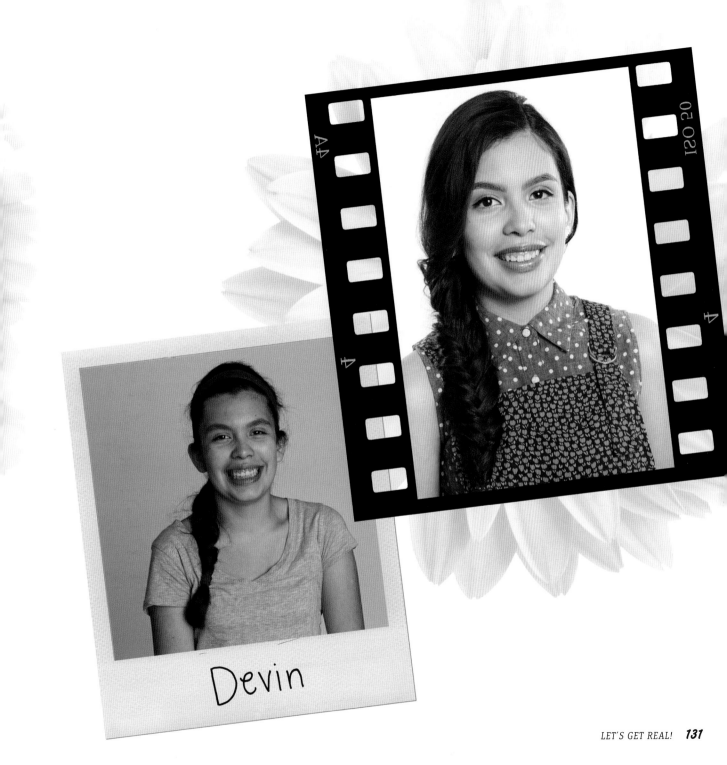

Devin

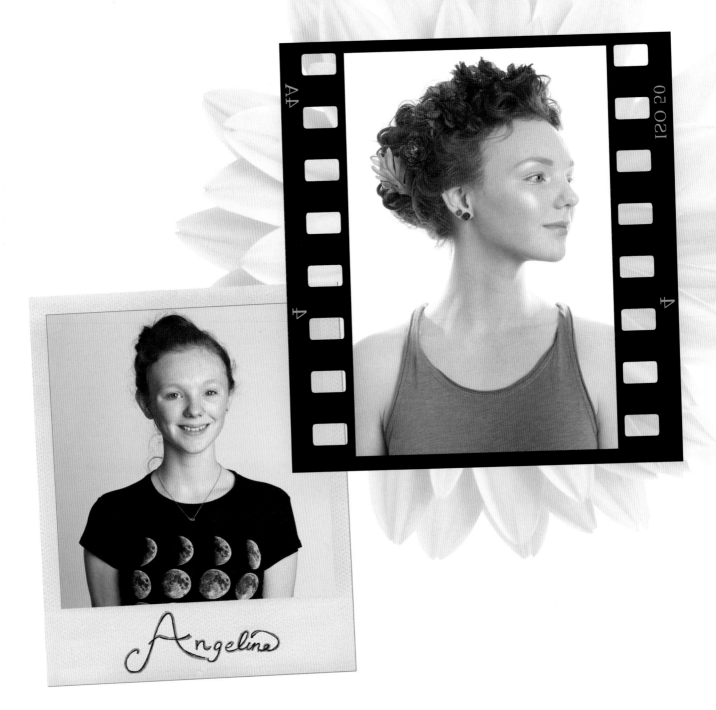

Angelina

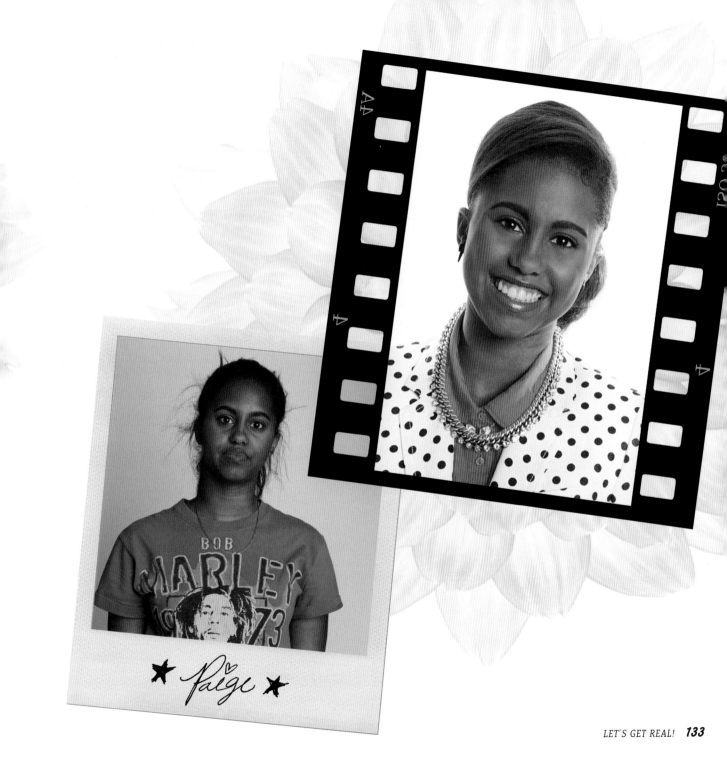

★ Paige ★

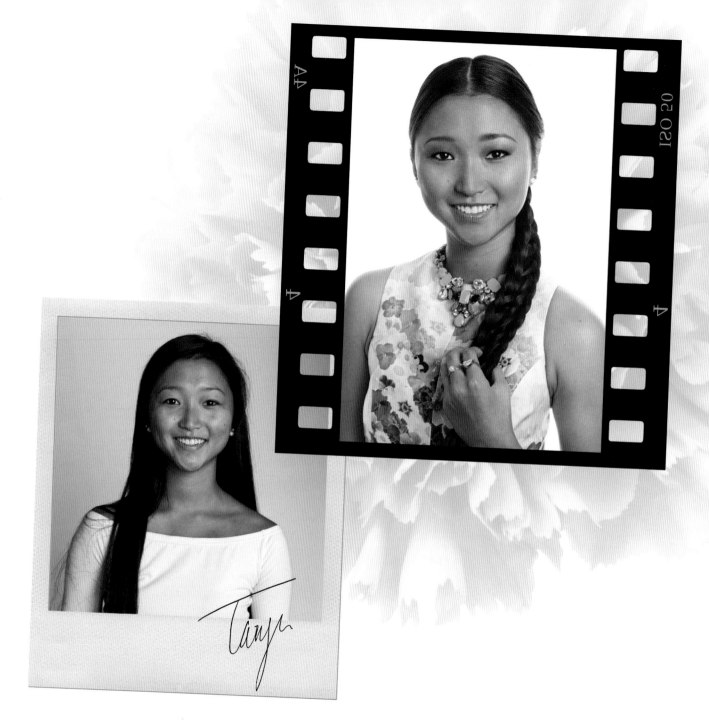

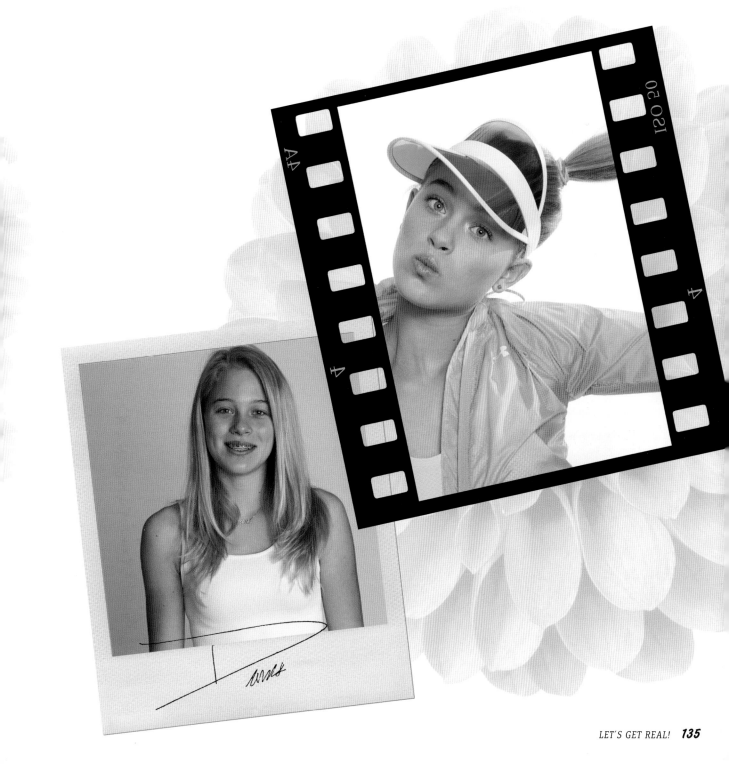

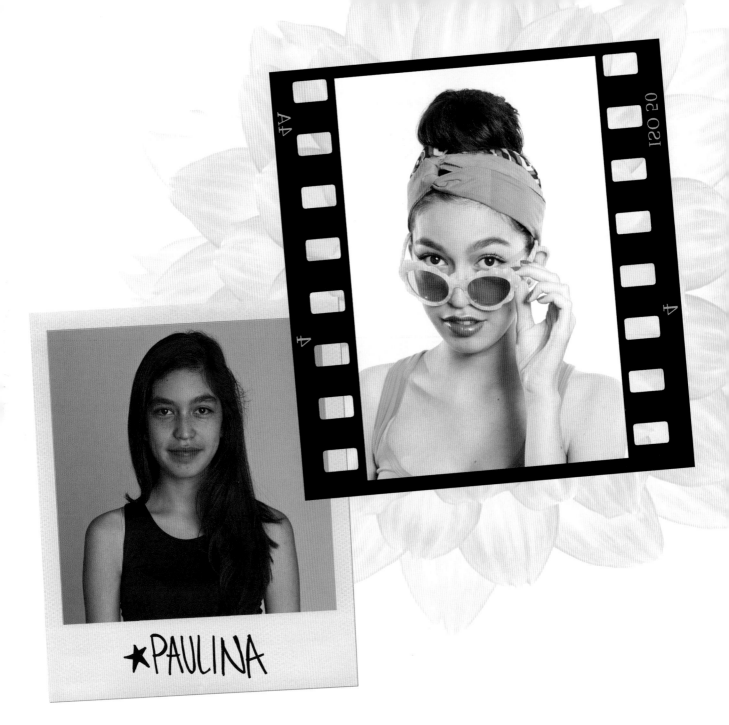

★PAULINA

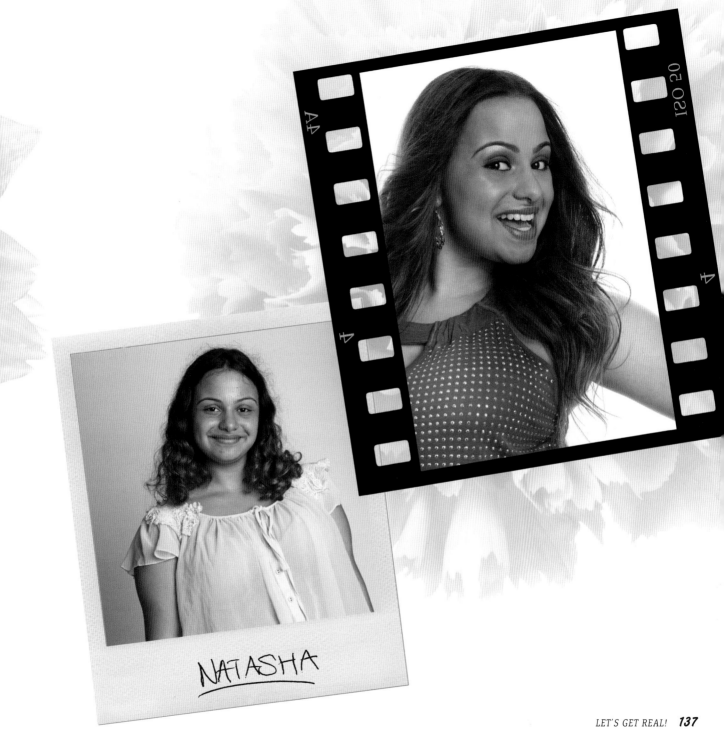

NATASHA

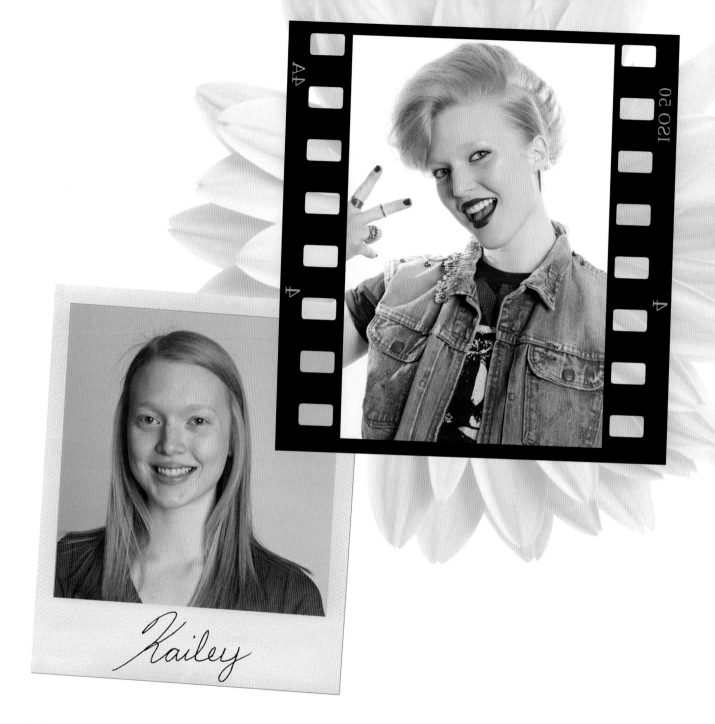

Kailey

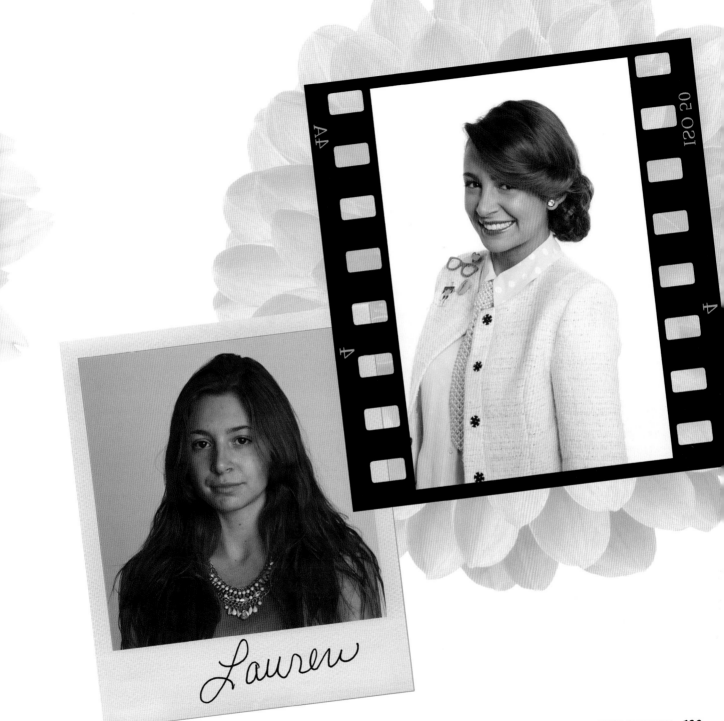

Lauren

Fresh
GROWN

Each and every girl featured on these pages exemplifies why I wanted to write this book in the first place. I am truly so inspired by all of the unique qualities that make teens special! Remember, any time you're feeling *less than*, reread Chapter 1, practice your Positive Mirror Mantras, and start spreading the seeds that are Contagious Compliments.

By supporting your fellow sisters, you're not only helping them out, you're building your own self-esteem as well. While I'm really excited that I could show you how to paint on the prettiest smoky eye and how to rock a red lip, what's really and truly important to me is that you cultivate your inner gardens—strong roots and soil will help you grow and bloom into the perfectly gorgeous flowers that you are, both inside and out. Of course, you know that you can always find me online: Twitter (@CarmindyBeauty), Facebook (Carmindy), Instagram (Carmindybeauty), and Tumblr (Carmindybeauty), so this conversation is far from over. In fact, it's just beginning!

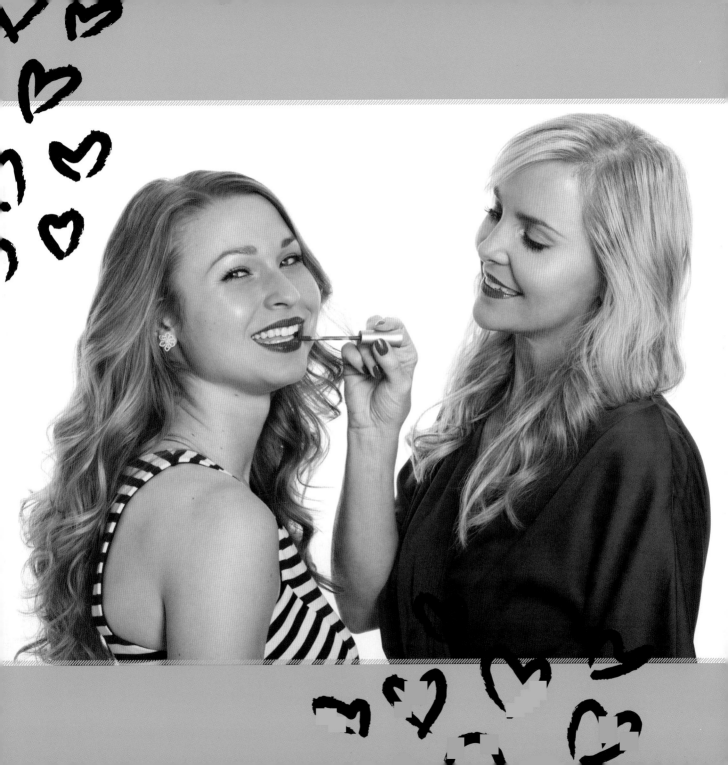

Acknowledgments

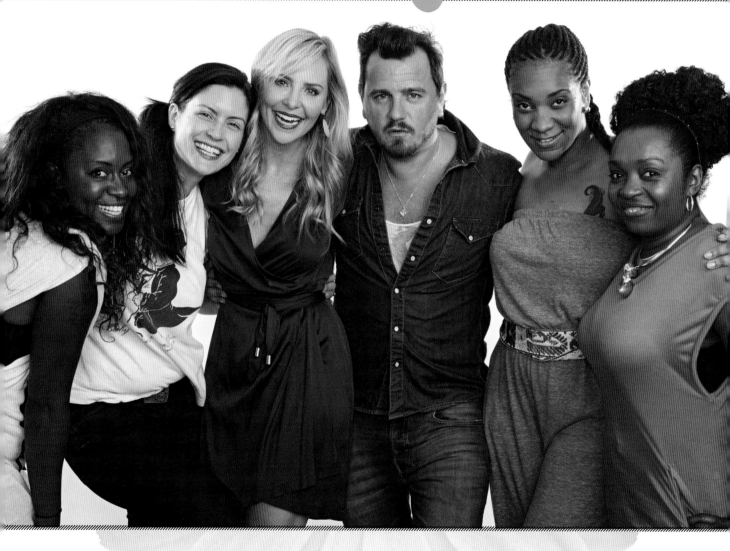

These hardworking and talented people all participated in *Bloom* and believe in its unlimited power. Thank you from the bottom of my heart for your tireless energy and passion in helping me teach teenage girls how to recognize their true blossoming beauty.

NATASHA MORA, PAULINA POLEYUMPTEWA, DEVIN JADE POLEYUMPTEWA, ANYA BERNSTEIN, ZHANÉ IRBY, DAVIS SILVER, LAUREN RUFFO, KAILEY DIEDRICK, MARISSA DIEDRICK, TARYN CHERUBINI, PAIGE BRYAN, and ANGELINA HOFFMAN—my lovely teen models that graced these pages with their blooming flower power. You blew my mind with your intelligence, grace, patience, and beauty.

JAY STERNBERG—where do I begin? You need a book-long dedication to your total belief in everything Carmindy, and without you I simply could not get it all done. You are my manager, agent, business partner, friend, and cheerleader. Your daily words of "It's all very positive" help me get through those crazy moments when I simply can't see it, but you are right, it always is!

EMILY SWEET and ABIGAIL KOONS—my powerhouse literary agents who got me from the moment we met. You guys rule!

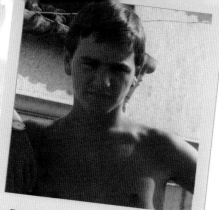

Daniel Garriga

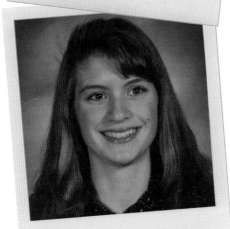

Chrissy Lloyd

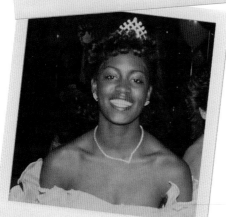

Merylin Mitchell

DANIEL GARRIGA—my photographer and videographer, who not only always makes me and my work look absolutely stunning but never says no to a project. Your devotion means the world to me.

JAI LENNARD—Daniel's supercool photo assistant— it was a blast to work with you.

DEVON JARVIS—the most incredible still-life photographer ever. Your shots are the baddest, boldest, and best!

SALVATORE COSENZA—a special thanks to a true artist and consummate professional.

CHRISSY LLOYD—stylist extraordinaire and the total fashion inspiration behind this book. Your artistic and creative vision brought these images to life and boosted the confidence of everyone who participated. You are pure joy!

LEAH KNOLL—hardworking stylist assistant to Chrissy. Thanks for the fun, stylish flavor you brought to the set each day.

MERYLIN MITCHELL—my fabulous key hairdresser, who always keeps the mood upbeat and fun. Not only can you rock a weave, but you also make the whole day a party and give from your heart like no other.

LISHL CLARK—hair stylist with magical hands, you whipped up the coolest dos in seconds and blew us all away with your talent.

CHANELLE MORRIS—hair assistant to Merylin and Lishl, who fully supported these two lovely ladies as they created amazing looks.

MYRDITH LEON-McCORMACK—nail artist to the stars, using her M2M damoreJon natural nail care line. You lovingly accepted this project without a moment's hesitation but also armed with the charge of empowerment.

VICTOR AMOS—Myrdith's fun assistant and innovative nail artist.

CHELSEA NETZBAND—for the beautiful floral head wreaths that made us all feel like goddesses.

HOLST & LEE JEWELRY—this insanely cool jewelry line was created by my fabulous friends Rochelle Lee and Natalie Holst and made my teens look chic and amazing.

LANNETTE PIERRE, HEATHER CONLAN, AND TARA CARRIGY—my great makeup assistants who hustled hard and had my back.

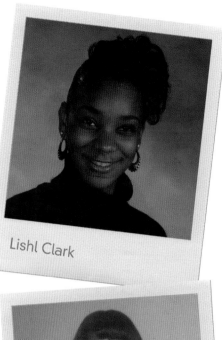

Lishl Clark

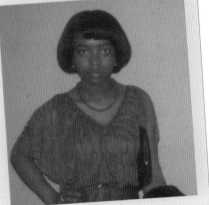

Myrdith Leon-McCormack

DANIELLE RUSSO—your work ethic and devotion as my personal assistant reminded me of myself when I was your age. I can't thank you enough for all your help and hard work. You symbolize the teens I am trying to reach, and you are a role model to your peers.

MARGHERITA RUSSO—thanks for being Danielle's other set of hands and for jumping right into the craziness with her.

THE KRAMER & KRAMER FAMILY: GAY FELDMAN, LESLIE KRAMER, AND FATIMA SCOTT—for keeping the machine running and the love coming.

KAROLINA HORN—my sweet little muse, you are a blessing in my life and shine with a light that inspires me to never forget the gold inside of us all.

GEOFFREY HORN—my king, you have showed me unlimited patience, honesty, encouragement, understanding, and more importantly, true love.

JACK, JULIE, QUINN, LISA, AND ELLARIE BOWYER—my supportive, awesome family! I love you so much.

About the Author

CARMINDY is a celebrated makeup artist known for her signature "Carmindizing" technique and her holistic approach that celebrates both inner and outer beauty. Millions of viewers counted on Carmindy to reveal the beauty of guests during the ten-year run of TLC's hit show *What Not to Wear*, where she played a key role in encouraging all women to embrace their true selves while showing them the tips and techniques of how to use makeup to highlight their best features. She is known for her upbeat and positive attitude, an attribute she carries into every aspect of her professional and personal lives.

Her work can be seen on the editorial pages of leading magazines such as *Cosmopolitan*; *Elle*; *InStyle*; *O, The Oprah Magazine*; *Essence*; *Self*; *Lucky*; *Seventeen*; *Marie Claire*; *Glamour*; and *Condé Nast Traveler*. In addition to writing three beauty books—*The 5-Minute Face*, *Get Positively Beautiful*, and *Crazy Busy Beautiful*—she created Carmindy & Co., a full range of beautiful color cosmetics that mirror her philosophy.

Through Twitter (@CarmindyBeauty), Facebook (Carmindy), and Instagram (@Carmindybeauty) she answers beauty questions and doles out advice to her fans. She also writes a beauty blog on Carmindy.com.

After spending her childhood in Southern California, Carmindy lived in Los Angeles, Milan, and Miami. Her lifelong passion for travel propelled her around the world, where she painted faces in Paris, on the beaches of Brazil, and in the streets of Havana. She now resides in New York City.

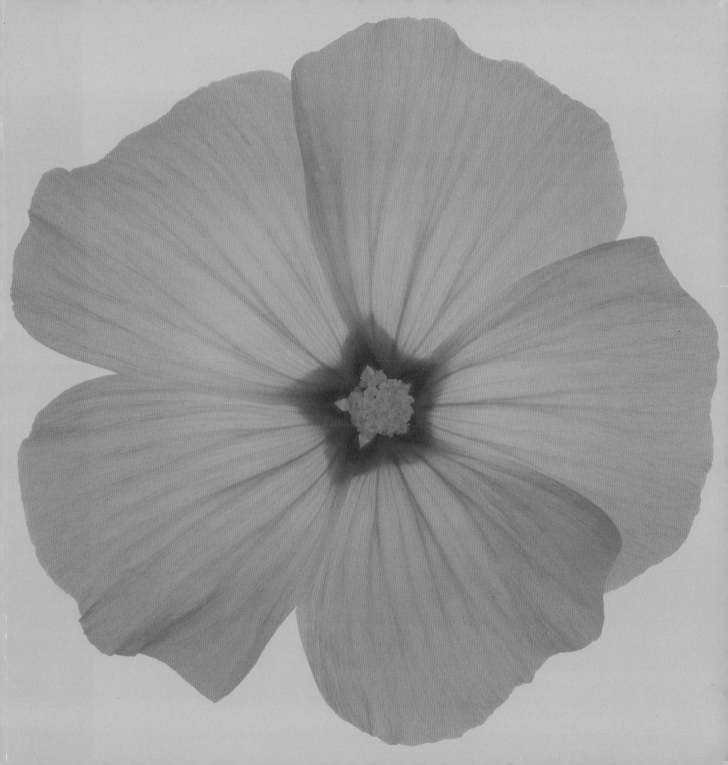

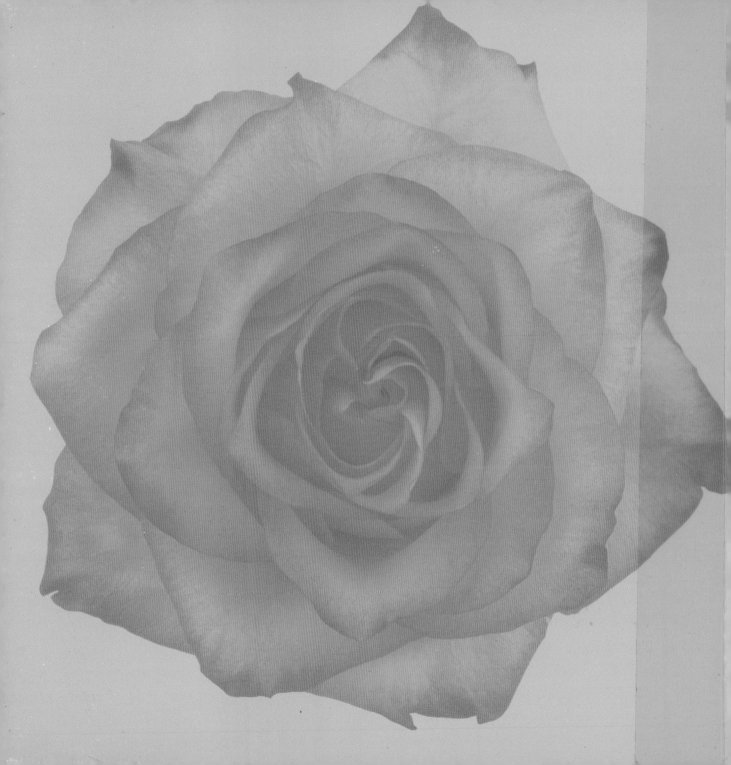